ETHICS C

Critical ad
international perspective

Edited by Marian Barnes, Tula Brannelly,
Lizzie Ward and Nicki Ward

First published in Great Britain in 2015 by

Policy Press
University of Bristol
1-9 Old Park Hill
Bristol
BS2 8BB
UK
t: +44 (0)117 954 5940
pp-info@bristol.ac.uk
www.policypress.co.uk

North America office:
Policy Press
c/o The University of Chicago Press
1427 East 60th Street
Chicago, IL 60637, USA
t: +1 773 702 7700
f: +1 773-702-9756
sales@press.uchicago.edu
www.press.uchicago.edu

© Policy Press 2015

British Library Cataloguing in Publication Data
A catalogue record for this book is available from the British Library

Library of Congress Cataloging-in-Publication Data
A catalog record for this book has been requested

ISBN 978-1-4473-1654-1 paperback
ISBN 978-1-4473-1651-0 hardcover
ISBN 978-1-4473-2333-4 ePub
ISBN 978-1-4473-2334-1 Kindle

The right of Marian Barnes, Tula Brannelly, Lizzie Ward and Nicki Ward to be identified as editors of this work has been asserted by them in accordance with the Copyright, Designs and Patents Act 1988.

Cover design by Hayes Design
Printed and bound in Great Britain by CMP, Poole
Policy Press uses environmentally responsible print partners

Together we dedicate this book to all those who have contributed to it. Thank you for making this task such an enjoyable one.

Contents

Acknowledgements

The editors would like to acknowledge all of those whom we have worked with and learnt from. To the service users, practitioner and academic colleagues, family members and friends whose contributions to our understanding of the ethics of care have convinced us of its importance – thank you!

Notes on contributors

Agnes Atim is an HIV care practitioner, activist and researcher. Agnes received her doctorate from the University of Reading, UK, and developed her current interest in the overlap between care, gender and conflict in the context of HIV as themes in research, policy and practice. She founded an international development and research organisation with a primary focus on care.

Marian Barnes is Emeritus Professor of Social Policy at the University of Brighton, UK. She previously held a chair in social research at the University of Birmingham and has also worked at the universities of Leeds and Sheffield. She is well known for her research in user involvement and user movements, public participation, citizenship and new forms of democratic practice. In the last few years her work has focused on the ethics of care, ageing and well-being. Her many publications include: *Power, Participation and Political Renewal* (Policy Press, with Janet Newman and Helen Sullivan); *Caring and Social Justice* (Palgrave); and *Care in Everyday Life* (Policy Press).

Amohia Boulton (Ngāti Ranginui, Ngai te Rangi, Ngāti Mutunga) is the Research Director at Whakauae Research for Māori Health and Development, a tribally owned and mandated research centre located in Whanganui, New Zealand. As a health services researcher Dr Boulton is concerned with the interface between national policies, planning practices and funding strategies for indigenous health services and the desires of local, indigenous communities for improving the health outcomes of their people. These interests have led to research and evaluation projects in traditional medicine, mental health, primary healthcare, public health and community-based health promotion.

Vivienne Bozalek has a PhD from Utrecht University. She is a professor of Social Work and the Director of Teaching and Learning at the University of the Western Cape, South Africa. Her areas of research and publications include the use of social justice and the political ethics of care perspectives, critical family studies, innovative pedagogical approaches in higher education, and feminist and participatory research methodologies. She has co-edited three books: *Community, Self and Identity: Educating South African Students for Citizenship*; *Discerning Hope in Educational Practices*; and *Activity Theory, Authentic Learning and Emerging Technologies: Towards a Transformative Higher Education Pedagogy*.

Tula Brannelly is a senior research fellow at the University of Surrey, UK, researching care, ethics and marginalised groups. Her research interests, developed while working in Aotearoa/New Zealand, include how care is shaped by political and structural influences and experienced by people who receive care, including the impacts of colonisation. Tula has a practice background in mental health and with older people. Her publications focus on the experience of care using an ethic of care analysis.

Diego de Merich is a teaching fellow at the London School of Economics and a Research Associate at the Institute for Intersectionality Research and Policy at Simon Fraser University, Canada. Researching in the areas of political theory, international development, deliberative democracy and critical feminist theory, his work on care ethics bridges recent findings on the neuroscience of human empathy with moral sentimentalist readings of sympathy and ethics. By foregrounding notions of empathy, empathic understanding, care and caring practices, his work seeks to highlight lacunae in traditional rights-based theories. In so doing, 'central capabilities' and practical ethics give way to the *practised* ethics (of context and relationship) long advocated by care theorists.

Ruth Evans is an associate professor in Human Geography at the University of Reading, UK. Her research focuses on caring relations, responses to death and gendered and intergenerational inequalities in access to land and other resources. Her publications include a co-authored book with Saul Becker, *Children Caring for Parents/Relatives with HIV/AIDS: Global Issues and Policy Responses* (2009, Policy Press) and articles on emotional interactions and an ethics of care in families affected by HIV (with Felicity Thomas, *Emotions, Space and Society*, 2009) and on sibling caregiving in youth-headed households orphaned by AIDS (*Area*, 2011; *Geoforum*, 2012; *African Journal of AIDS Research*, 2012).

Ann Fudge Schormans is an associate professor in the School of Social Work at McMaster University (Hamilton, Ontario, Canada). A practising social worker for many years, she worked with people with intellectual disabilities (ID) in the community living and child welfare sectors. Employing inclusive, co-researcher methodologies and knowledge production, along with arts-informed methods, her current research interests include an exploration of the use of city space by people labelled ID; the intersection of ID with education, employment and experiences of homelessness; the parenting experiences and aspirations of people with ID; and the friendships and social inclusion of youth with ID.

Anne Liveng is an associate professor affiliated to the Center for Health Promotion Research at Roskilde University, Denmark. Her primary research interests are in elderly care, learning in health and care work and policies regarding the healthcare sector. She applies a psycho-social approach in theory and methods and is inspired by critical theory and care ethics. In her current work she focuses on equality, equity and intersectional perspectives in connection to health and care. She is a member of International Research Group for Psycho-Societal Analysis (www.irgfpsa.org) and the Nordic Network for Health Promotion Research (www.nhv.se).

Teodora Manea studied Philosophy (1992–96) and completed her PhD (2002) at the 'Al.I Cuza' University of Iasi, Romania. She worked at the same university (as a senior lecturer, 2000–09) and had a fruitful collaboration with several prestigious German universities. Since 2010 she has been working for the University of Exeter Medical School, UK, teaching medical humanities and medical sociology. She works as an ethics expert for the European Commission and does medical interpreting. Her recent publications include 'Medical Bribery and the Ethics of Trust', *Journal of Medicine and Philosophy* (2015, 40(1): 26-43) and 'Our Posthuman Skin Condition', in *Handbook of Posthumanism in Film and* Television (Palgrave Macmillan, 2015).

Ingunn Moser is a professor and rector in Diakonhjemmet University College, Oslo, Norway, and adjunct professor in the Centre for Technology, Innovation and Culture, University of Oslo. She has published extensively on disability, subjectivity and embodiment in relation to new technologies. Her more recent research focuses on cultures of caring, dementia care and uses of telecare technologies in the care for the old.

Anke Niehof studied social anthropology and demography. Her PhD thesis was entitled 'Women and Fertility in Madura, Indonesia' (1985, Leiden University). For 20 years she headed the Chair Group of the Sociology of Consumption and Households at Wageningen University, the Netherlands. Since April 2013, she has been Professor Emeritus. She publishes on the household production of food security, well-being and care, women's reproductive health, and the impacts of HIV/AIDS on women and food and livelihood systems in sub-Saharan Africa, using gender and actor-oriented approaches.

Laura Steckley is a senior lecturer at the University of Strathclyde in Glasgow, Scotland. Her research interests are primarily focused on residential childcare/child and youth care. She has published extensively on physical restraint, as well as wider areas of theory and practice in working with young people who have experienced trauma and other difficulties. Laura's forthcoming publications include a co-authored book, *Creating a Healing Home: Using the Everyday to Recover from Loss and Pain* (Jessica Kingsley), and findings from an exploratory study on threshold concepts in residential childcare/child and youth care (CELCIS).

Hilde Thygesen is an occupational therapist and has a PhD in Sociology. Currently she is working as an associate professor at the Institute of Nursing and Health at Diakonhjemmet University College in Oslo, Norway. The focus of her research is on care practices, with a particular interest in the relations between care and technology, and in normative issues. Her publications relate to empirical ethics and the use of telecare technologies in the care for the old.

Joan Tronto is a professor of Political Science at the University of Minnesota, USA. Her research interests in political theory include the ethic of care and postcolonial political theory. Tronto has published over 40 essays and two main books: *Moral Boundaries: A Political Argument for an Ethic of Care* (1993) and *Caring Democracy: Markets, Equality and Justice* (2013).

Lizzie Ward is a senior research fellow in the School of Applied Social Science at the University of Brighton, UK. Lizzie is a qualitative researcher and her research interests include: age and ageing, care ethics, participatory research and experiential knowledge, gender and feminist methodologies. She works in the field of community-based participatory research and has a particular interest in co-production and working with older people as co-researchers. She has published in the areas of applying care ethics to research practice and social care practice with older people.

Nicki Ward is a lecturer in the School of Social Policy at the University of Birmingham, UK. Her research and teaching interests coalesce around issues relating to care, ethics and values and diversity.

Nicki is particularly interested in intersectional identities and the practice of care and this is the focus of her publications. Nicki is a qualified social worker and has a practice background working with people with learning disabilities.

Section One
Conceptual and theoretical developments

ONE

Introduction: the critical significance of care

Marian Barnes, Tula Brannelly, Lizzie Ward and Nicki Ward

In the 22 years since Joan Tronto's ground-breaking work *Moral Boundaries* (Tronto, 1993), arguments for a political ethic of care have spread far and wide – both literally in a geographical sense and in the many different contexts in which its core ideas have been taken up. Central to the development of a distinctive ethical perspective built around the significance of care in all our lives is the understanding that humans are relational beings. We do not start out as autonomous individuals who have to seek to make relationships with others. Rather, our survival from birth is dependent on the care we receive from others. Our development requires others to nurture this and throughout our lives we need relationships with others as a basis on which we can grow, learn and experience well-being. Our identity is generated substantially through how others see and respond to us, rather than emerging solely from within ourselves. Most of us seek someone or some people with whom we can share our lives. And for all of us there are times when illness or emotional or physical frailty mean that we need the care, help and support of others to enable us to deal with everyday life. For some people and at some stages of life the need for regular, intimate and skilled care is a necessity for effective functioning and even survival.

Care ethics is based in this relational ontology. From its early articulation by Gilligan (1982) as a different way of thinking about right judgements from those deriving from justice ethics, through a 'feminine' perspective on ethics and moral education (Noddings, 1984) to the explicitly 'feminist' and political work inspired by *Moral Boundaries*, the ethics of care has countered an ethical perspective that starts from abstract moral reasoning and that assumes that we start out as disconnected individuals who then have to seek to form relationships. This is the basis for its attraction to those working in the social sciences, including those working in applied spheres such as social work and nursing, as well as to moral philosophers who recognise the importance of grounding moral theory within real lives. From the perspective of moral philosophy, Walker (2007) has argued that:

> Morality arises and goes on between people, recruiting human capacities for self-awareness and awareness of others' awareness; for feeling and learning to feel particular things in response to what one is aware of; for expressing judgement and feeling in the responses appropriate to them. (Walker, 2007, p 5)

From a social science perspective Andrew Sayer also argues for a 'breaking of the boundaries' between social science and philosophy. On the basis that 'The most important questions people tend to face in their everyday lives are normative ones of what is good or bad about what is happening to them, including how others are treating them, and of how to act, and what to do for the best' (Sayer, 2011, p 1), social science needs to be capable of engaging with the centrality of the ways in which what we value impacts on what we do and how we relate to others.

The ethics of care, then, can and has been applied to diverse relationships that constitute everyday lives, professional practices, the analysis of social and public policies and international relations, and the design of the physical environments in which diverse encounters with others take place. No collection of essays such as this one can encompass the full range of contexts that can benefit from a critical analysis from the perspective of care ethics. In an editorial introducing two special issues of *Ethics and Social Welfare* Christine Koggel and Joan Orme (2010) argue that the diversity of work on care ethics illustrates its applicability to all aspects of human relations and organisation. The contributions to the present collection illustrate and develop important aspects of this diversity, demonstrating the significance of care ethics as a transformative way of viewing social relations within and beyond those contexts usually defined by reference to 'care'. In this introduction we consider both the power and the importance of this perspective.

Care ethics: personal and political

In her recent book, *Caring Democracy. Markets, Equality and Justice*, Tronto (2013) has developed the political character of feminist care ethics. Arguing that 'democratic political life has to be about *something*' (p ix), her starting point is that democratic politics should be about how we think about caring in its broadest sense and how we allocate responsibilities for ensuring this. For Tronto the democratic deficit and the care deficit are linked. To resolve one requires working on the other:

> Democratic politics should center upon assigning responsibilities for care, and for ensuring that democratic citizens are as capable as possible of participating in the assignment of these responsibilities. (Tronto, 2013, p 7)

This position continues her radical undermining of the moral boundaries that have sought to separate the private world in which care happens 'naturally' from the political world in which issues of security, economics, work and international relations are thought of as unconnected to the personal and interpersonal concerns of care giving and receiving, and both can be separated from abstract, universalist musings on 'the good life'. This political as well as ethical and personal engagement with the significance of care in all our lives distinguishes feminist care ethics from other ways of thinking about care. The transformations that care ethics seek are not solely that care provided face to face will be 'better', but that care thinking will impact on the way we think about politics and the way political decisions are reached. Such decisions affect the possibility for 'good care' by impacting the resources available to, and institutional cultures within which, hands-on care is provided, and reflect ideological positions, in particular the belief in markets as appropriate mechanisms through which to 'deliver' care. Sevenhuijsen's (2003) argument that policy analysis from the perspective of care ethics should not be limited to analysis, but should also propose ways in which such policies might be 'renewed', reflects this transformative ambition.

In her more recent work, Tronto explores a number of key issues that have become particularly salient in the years since *Moral Boundaries* was published and which are evident in the arguments developed through contributions to this collection. One is the relationship between care and justice. Gilligan's (1982) distinction of an ethic of care from an ethic of justice was vital to naming care thinking as distinct from the abstract moral reasoning underpinning justice ethics. Some versions of care ethics have argued that justice cannot be integrated with care. Others have moved beyond this divide between care and justice to explore the significance of each to the other (for example Hankivsky, 2004; Barnes, 2006; Held, 2006; Barnes and Brannelly, 2008; Tronto, 2013). Tronto argues that *caring with* 'requires that caring needs and the ways in which they are met need to be consistent with democratic commitments to justice, equality and freedom for all' (Tronto, 2013, p 23).

Bringing care and justice together requires focusing on collective as well as individual responsibilities for care. 'Privileged irresponsibility' refers to the way powerful people do not recognise their own need for care and consequently fail to think that care is anything to do with them. Tronto (2013) identifies different 'get out passes' that are used to deny responsibility for care. The first of these is the 'protection pass'. Protection is a gendered construct and, to put it crudely, men do the protection while women care. However, Tronto also argues that some protection can be considered as care. For example, she suggests renewing prisons as places of care rather than punishment. Second is the 'production pass'. Men provide the pay cheque, women do the hands-on care. The production pass in the renewed democracy does not allow the holder to 'get out of care'. This expands the activities of care to those who currently accept no responsibility for it. Care for 'only my own' is also critiqued, as it activates the resources of those most able to provide them, thereby missing out the caring for people who need resources most. Finally, Tronto highlights the need for a renewed economic regulation that understands the provision of care beyond the passes of 'charity and bootstraps' for people who most require it. Again, Tronto argues that these activities need to be understood as care.

Global care and justice

A political ethic of care requires an international and global perspective. One aspect of the uneven processes of economic globalisation and of changing demographics is the increasing visibility and significance of the global movement of care labour – necessary to sustain care deficits in the West, and, some have argued, building care deficits elsewhere (Mahon and Robinson, 2011). While evidence suggests that we need to develop a nuanced understanding of the impact of migration on the way in which care is practised by transnational families, rather than assuming that migration inevitably fractures care relationships (Parrenas, 2005; Zontini, 2013), it is nevertheless the case that care migration has generated new ethical as well as political and personal challenges. The implications of these shifts, for those who are migrating as well as for those left behind in the countries of origin, highlight another set of issues connected to the impossibilities of viewing social justice solely within the boundaries of nation-states. Mahon and Robinson (2011, p 25) argued that the movement of care labour from poorer countries to the US and Europe has 'translated the unequal relations of personal interdependency into the unequal relations of transnational interdependency'. At an interpersonal level there is evidence of difficult and sometimes abusive relationships between migrant care workers with little power and those who are dependent on personal care for their survival (Cangiano et al, 2009; Nare, 2013). These complex interdependencies in the context of unequal power relationships in which 'race', nationality, gender, age, disability and socioeconomic status intersect, emphasise the necessity of thinking about care and justice together.

Another ethical and political issue brought into focus by a global perspective on care concerns the way we treat those forced by violence and oppression to seek asylum in another country. This challenges our sense of responsibility to care for strangers or unknown others (Barnes, 2012a, ch 6). Traditional understandings of care have emphasised this as something practised in intimate contexts, between people who are known to each other personally or via professional roles as care givers. While most might accept, in line with Engster (2007), that our responsibilities for care vary with the degree of 'closeness' to those in need, a political ethic of care that emphasises collective as well as individual responsibilities draws attention to the importance of care for strangers (see Young, 2011 for a related analysis from a 'justice' perspective). A greater awareness of the interconnectedness of humanity across national boundaries as well as within interpersonal networks requires a politics and practices that encompass care and justice well beyond 'face to face' care.

Care ethics and the historical moment – the failure of neoliberalism

The limits of liberal individualism within a marketised model of health and welfare are exposed by the movements of care labour and the dilemmas these generate. Recent years have witnessed multiple evidences of the failures of neoliberalism – and not only for care. The penetration of marketised models within health and welfare – based on 'contractual relationships between self-interested strangers of equal standing' (Lloyd, 2012, p 5) is understood as *the* desired form of public service. But these assumptions do not reflect the realities of unequal relationships that have particular significance in relation to care. Taking an international perspective on health and care for older people, Lloyd links care migration with the developing emphasis on individual consumption of care services:

global socioeconomic inequalities are inextricably linked with the micro-context of care. Older people in high income countries might be able to exercise choice to have personalised services in their own homes, but their choice is made possible by the migration of low-paid workers from low and middle income countries to carry out the work. The capacity of the ethics of care to draw the links between the micro and macro levels of care is of particular importance in revealing the global nature of caring work. (Lloyd, 2012, p 136)

The assumptions that underpin hegemonic neoliberalism – that all aspects of human life can be organised on market principles: choice, consumption and, above all, the prioritising of the individual as a free agent making rational choices and consuming within the market, filter down, and through, social and welfare policies at all levels. These are not uniform processes, and as they interact with different welfare regimes and historically developed conditions they have produced unevenly spread inequalities between and within nation-states. Yet the overarching frame of neoliberalism has fundamentally shaped relationships between citizens and states in relation to responsibilities, welfare and citizenship. This affects the ways welfare services are constructed, the way the 'welfare subject' is thought about, and the way development is conceived and practised at international level.

Neoliberalism has been under attack in the wake of the 2008 banking meltdown and financial crisis. The guilty bankers and traders were, after all, taking the 'principle' of profit above all else to the limit. This brought questions about values back to public consciousness, as Baggini (2012, online) remarked, 'making morality fashionable again'. He argued that after decades of self-interest, the economic crash and public outcry at governmental responses to banking scandals, including the loss of welfare jobs and services, created an opportunity for morality to recover a political dimension. The desire for alternative visions was apparent in angry public responses to austerity measures as well as a renewed interest in solidarity and mutuality coming from some academic and policy quarters (for example, Allen, 2013). This has been reflected for some time in communitarian discourses expressing the need for a more cooperative civil society. Communitarianism has attracted advocates across the political spectrum in the UK and the US. In the UK it is evident in recent claims for the Left to 'rediscover' the values of mutuality and reciprocity. Others have argued for faith-based approaches as a response to what is perceived to be a moral crisis in civil and political life fuelled by excessive individualism (see, for example, Beaumont and Cloke, 2012; Jawad, 2012).

But the crisis did not just prompt questions of public morality and a resurgence of interest in ideals of community and mutuality. Davies (2012) questioned whether the banking crisis would spark a paradigm shift in economic policy making. Certainly this crisis questioned the core tenets of (neo)liberalism – the privileging of the market as the main arbiter of public choice and efficiency – and the role of the state in facilitating these without taking a 'moral' stance on what choices (or preferences) might be understood as 'good' or 'bad'. Communitarianism proposes a conception of the individual as a social being constituted by shared values and relationships with others. However, suggestions that this means communitarianism can be equated with feminist care ethics have been rebutted (for example, Kittay, 2001a), and Davies (2012) argues that the emergent 'neo-communitarian' critique reflects a 'policy technocrat' position informed by behavioural and happiness economics.

Thus the ethic of care now has to engage with the underlying assumptions of this neocommunitarian paradigm that is becoming part of the orthodoxy within public policy. Davies argues that neocommunitarianism and behavioural economics do not replace neoliberalism; rather, behavioural interventions aim 'to teach and encourage people how to behave in a more rational, coherent fashion, precisely to enable the *survival* of neoliberalism' (Davies, 2012, p 775).

The 'austerity measures' that wealthier, most often Western, nations enacted as a response to the global economic crisis entailed cuts in care services and in welfare entitlements impacting on the most marginalised and vulnerable people (Levitas, 2012). In less wealthy countries, public spending remains at a minimum, with an emphasis on charitable giving, despite economic gains that have widened gaps of inequality as in, for example, New Zealand. Deficit-reduction programmes that centre on large cuts in public expenditure are impacting unevenly within and between (European Union) countries, not only leading to severe material consequences for those who are most vulnerable, but also forcing 'efficiency' drives in service provision. This translates on the ground into the ways in which care services are commissioned and provided within a framework of minimum costs set against measurable outcomes.

Before the impact of financial crisis and austerity, policy in the UK and Western Europe had emphasised cash-for-care schemes that enable service users to decide on and purchase their own 'care services'. Such schemes are an obvious example of the embedding of market philosophy within the design, provision and delivery of welfare services. Evidence for the 'success' of such policies is mixed (for example, Grootegoed, 2013; Moran et al, 2013), but more important for this discussion is the need to consider the broad implications of this way of accessing services in terms of the political, democratic and ethical significance of care as a collective responsibility. Barnes (2011) offered one critique of the UK approach to 'personalisation' from an ethic of care perspective. Her analysis suggested that this may undermine collective responsibility for care:

> Adoption of this approach also has implications for collective responsibilities for unknown others. What will be the consequences of the widespread adoption of a model of individual service commissioning for the preparedness of those able to assert 'privileged irresponsibility' to commit to ensure public funding of high-quality welfare provision? (Barnes, 2011, p 165)

Market building is both an objective of cash-for-care schemes and a requirement for their success. However, there is little evidence in the UK that community-based services are developing to provide the sort of options for support that service users might choose (Needham, 2014). In fact, small user-led services are at risk because of the removal of grant funding (Rose et al, 2013). This is unsurprising in view of the combined policy objectives of reducing costs at the same time as 'empowering' service users. So, are markets incompatible with care?

Tronto's (2013) response to this question is formulated in the context of an American system in which the market has had a much bigger role than in European welfare states – many of which are fast seeking to emulate the US model. Much of her analysis is familiar to those who have critiqued the emergence of market-based approaches to welfare in the UK and Western Europe since the late 1980s. But the necessity to reiterate such critiques offers an important reminder of the fundamental problems of market thinking in an era where such critiques have become obscured, and in a context in which 'responsibility' has become located in individual obligations to behave in acceptable ways, rather than the responsibilities of states to enable care for citizens. The power of market discourse is evident in the way that arguments for justice and recognition are being framed in the language of finance and economics. For example, in making the case for the recognition due to unpaid care givers, Carers UK reports that carers save the economy £87 billion a year, while £5.3 billion is lost to the economy by carers giving up work to care.[1] Other groups seeking social justice are also forced to make a business case for diversity.

Tronto's discussion of care, markets and justice considers the relational qualities of human nature and the temporal dimensions of this. A reliance on market thinking obscures the prospect of seeing how social structures create and perpetuate inequality: 'Citizens are not equal by virtue of being declared equal, but through an elaborate social process through which they become equal' (Tronto, 2013, p 120). Markets are oriented to the future rather than the past and do not consider past injustices that have created harm. Those who are victims of such harm, such as people subject to racism, are castigated for not standing up for themselves and asserting their own needs and choices. But this is hard to do when you have been harmed. Care always has a past and how we respond to past injustices is one of the largest ethical questions we need to face.

This has an especial significance for a global perspective on care and care ethics. The argument for acknowledging the past in the present in order to care for the future is particularly pertinent in colonised societies. Such societies share three characteristics. The first is that political, cultural and social change has occurred as a result of colonisation; the second is that colonisation has resulted in social and political inequality; and the third is that indigenous values are different to those of colonisers. Land loss and dispossession, population decimation (Durie, 2001) and denial of indigenous knowledge (Smith, 1999) – what Visvanathan (2005) has described as an absence of 'cognitive justice' – have impacted to differing degrees in different nations, dependent on the timing and processes of colonisation. But the devaluing of indigenous knowledge and values that are grounded in humanness and the importance of connection is a consequence of Western imperialism across the globe. Such values are being reasserted. The African concept of Ubuntu; *suma qamaña*, a collective concept of well-being that was adopted as a central value in the Bolivian constitution of 2009; and the Māori principles of whānaungatanga or relationship building all share an affinity with care ethics and offer a challenge to the rational individualism dominating Western thinking.

Justice, renewal and virtue

We have argued that a political ethic of care inevitably focuses the relationship between care and justice. Sevenhuijsen's (2003) inclusion of a process of 'renewal' within policy analysis from an ethic of care, as well as Tronto's recent work on renewing democracy, emphasise its transformational potential.

Some have considered care ethics to be a form of virtue ethics (such as Halwani, 2003). But we suggest that this ignores this critical and transformational potential. The characteristics of virtue ethics are present, by and large, in the integrity of care as described by Tronto (1993). The four cardinal ethical virtues of temperance, justice, courage and practical wisdom associated with ancient ethics were further expanded by Christian philosophers in the Middle Ages to include the theological virtues of faith, hope and charity or love (Honderich 1995). Current virtues include compassion, respect, dignity and care. Tronto's (1993) integrity of care principles of attentiveness, competence, responsibility and responsiveness incorporate virtues such as respect, dignity and openness to the other's position. Care requires that people practise with compassion, respect, and treat people with dignity. The achievement of justice would also feature as part of the moral good. There may have been a moment when care ethics were described in terms of an intimate relationship where the virtues are played out, as in Nel Nodding's work (1984). However, virtue ethics remains a moral philosophy, focused on becoming and being a 'good' person, whereas care ethics aims for political as well as personal renewal.

Others who are concerned to improve the practice of care have suggested synthesis between care ethics and other aspects of care and ethics, such as narrative ethics of care (Paulsen, 2011). Here care ethics is dissected and the principles of integrity of care are separated from the broader philosophy of care ethics. While this may be because the principles provide an accessible framework to guide care practices, the separation of care ethics from the broader philosophical standpoint serves to depoliticise the question of how to improve care. The critical feminist political position in which care ethics is based makes it more than a set of characteristics for the pursuit of good; it is a broad set of theories for the pursuit of justice that require action within political and institutional systems as well as within interpersonal caring relationships. This becomes particularly significant when we come to consider both the origins of and responses to abuse and poor practice in 'care' settings.

The crisis of and for care

Personal or professional characteristics or virtues alone do not achieve justice. They may not achieve care. In a healthcare setting, each profession has a set of rules or a code of conduct that sets the standards by which the people in their care may be treated. These are usually virtues based, such as preservation of dignity and respect. But still there are broader political contexts within which practice occurs, in terms both of the institutional culture and societal norms that impact on care. Bowden (2000) has considered the significance of this in the context of healthcare and Ash (2010) in relation to elder care. The failures of systems that do not prioritise care as a value and practice were evident in the Francis Inquiry into unusually high incidences of death in Stafford Hospital, England. The report opened with the following statement:

> [I]t should be patients – not numbers – which counted. That remains my view. The demands for financial control, corporate governance, commissioning and regulatory systems are understandable and in many cases necessary. But it is not the system itself which will ensure that the patient is put first day in and day out. Any system should be capable of caring and delivering an acceptable level of care to each patient treated ... (Francis, 2013, p 5)

Where abuse occurs, individuals who should be 'caring' may be seen as shifting from the moral to the immoral, or turning to the dark side, a part of human nature where good cannot be continually maintained. But it would be wrong to account for abuse solely by reference to evil deeds or evil people. The accounts contained within the Francis Inquiry do not just suggest a failed moral compass of some practitioners, but significantly point to systemic tolerance of poor practice. It was the complaints of family and friends, not professionals. that finally highlighted the serious shortcomings that prompted this Inquiry.

Abuse and poor care in settings designed to ensure care have a long and disturbing history. One factor that is salient in the poor treatment of people in different contexts is the marginalisation of groups of people judged as having less social worth: those with learning disabilities, with mental health problems or dementia, for example (Gilmour and Brannelly, 2010; Kittay and Carlson, 2010; Brannelly 2011). Conventional approaches to evidence of maltreatment are to assert human and civil rights that need to be upheld so as to ensure procedural justice. However, rights-based approaches are unable to provide justice for groups of people who are the most marginalised, and sometimes the most vulnerable. Kittay's (1999) work brings to bear her insights as a feminist, as the mother of a daughter with cognitive disabilities and as a philosopher to critique liberal notions of justice in this context.

But there *is* a need both to account for abusive practice and to explore and explain care practices that have been experienced as oppressive and thus the source of a critique of care per se. Contributors to this book consider care practices that have the potential to deliver care and justice. Understanding the context and practices of care is important to understanding the difficulties and complexity of messy care situations in order to know what citizens require in the way of care.

The success of the disability movement in challenging notions of care and care practices, in demanding a rethinking of 'care' from the perspectives of care receivers and in arguments for justice and recognition based on rights has had a profound effect on the development of services and also on the valuing of the notion of care in policy (Barnes, 2012a). Care has been conceptualised in different ways at different times and has been subject to a number of different discursive constructions. However, it has tended to be associated with the physical act of care or nurturing, and thus with supporting people to meet their basic physiological needs for food, warmth, personal care and mobility. This equation of care with the need for support, and consequently with a deficit – the inability to care for oneself – has contributed to the relegation of care to the private sphere and has constructed it as a private activity through which one person (the care giver) tends to the needs of another (the care receiver). From a care ethics perspective this obscures and marginalises notions of interdependence and the need that we all have for care. For many within the disability rights movement, this construction of care and the care relationship is what creates relationships of power and dependency. Care in this sense has been experienced as paternalistic, demeaning and disempowering. Care as a concept has become devalued and seen as synonymous with dependency. The very word care has now been replaced in many policy contexts with concepts such as support and enablement, which are seen to be more representative of independence and self-determination than 'care'.

Like other claims for rights made within the liberal paradigm (for example, those for 'women's rights'), the call of the disability rights movement for justice, rights and self-determination has readily been absorbed into liberal discourses, rather than fundamentally challenging their basis. Policies for welfare provision to those needing care and support have responded to claims for greater control and involvement through the promotion of consumerist strategies. Recent policies have translated this into self-directed support, a predominantly financial initiative that promises the individual greater control to buy the support they need (Barnes, 2011). In addition, a view of autonomy as individual self-sufficiency and economic independence – the ability to participate in the workforce – drives activation policies in many Western welfare states (Clarke, 2005; Darmon and Perez, 2011).

Arguably, this has played into the hands of those who equate activation with a step back from state responsibilities. More positively, this has added impetus to development of the 'responsiveness' principle in care ethics and to focusing greater attention on the active role of care receiver in the processes and relationships within care. One aspect of this is to recognise the importance of the experiential knowledge of care receivers to enabling care (Barnes, 2012a).

Challenges from disability activists reflect wider shifts in theorising about knowledge claims and, in particular, power and voice in knowledge production. Alongside this are developments in the theorisation of gender, ethnicity and sexuality, moving beyond a focus on difference and towards the ways in which different aspects of identity and social location interact through the paradigm of intersectionality (Yuval-Davis, 2006a; Anthias, 2013). Among other things this has called into question assumptions that care is a dyadic, one-way process, making the two distinct categories of 'care giver' and 'care receiver' unsustainable (Ward, 2011). Relationships of care, whether between individuals (the carer and the cared for) or between individuals and the state, are embedded within (and embedded with) different relationships of power.

The activity of care, as discussed earlier, has been conceptualised as an individual relationship between two people where one is defined as the care giver and the other the care receiver. Williams (2012) notes that policies freeze identities into either care giver or care receiver. In this way policy both creates and reinforces a discourse of dependence and independence; it is not possible to be both carer and cared for at the same time, and individuals have to position themselves in one or other way in order to access services and support. This reification of roles within caring relationships obscures the complexity of individual identity and ignores the intersectionality of people's experience.

The ethics of care encourages a view of care as an activity interpreted, viewed and enacted through particular people negotiating caring in specific socio-cultural contexts, in which they are exploring the right thing to do for themselves and their relationships (Williams, 2004a). It is in this sense that care is seen as a dynamic relationship, formed between those helping and those needing help (Folgheraiter, 2007). This then emphasises notions not of independence but of interdependence or relational autonomy (MacKenzie and Stoljar, 2000). And it encourages recognition of both the embedded nature of caring relationships and the range of people involved in these. Care ethics emphasises the everyday nature of caring relationships in all lives, where everyone needs care. Kittay noted:

> If each is worthy of care then the caregiver too, deserves care ... Even as I care for another, I, too, am worthy of care. This is [a] notion of fairness and reciprocity that is not dyadic but one that involves at least a third party, and more properly an infinite spiral of relationships. (Kittay, 2001a, p 536)

Williams (2012) argues for care to be valued as a social good. What care ethics provides is a way of viewing and analysing care, reclaiming not only the language of care but also the practice, within a philosophical and ideological frame within which care is seen as an act of citizenship that embraces both the personal and the political.

The 'crisis' for care is also linked to demographic change and the increase in population ageing. The expected rise in the need for care services, together with concern that there will be fewer economically active working-age people, has contributed to a powerful discourse of active ageing, making its presence felt at various levels from economically driven labour market policies to the promotion of consumerist life-style choices (Lloyd, 2012).

The policy response to global ageing is underpinned by assumptions that by promoting 'active ageing' and independence (WHO, 2002) while keeping the costs of care under tight control (spending cuts in health and care, restructuring of services), the 'crisis' can be managed. The numbers of people living into older age have likewise led to debates surrounding a future 'care deficit' based on fairly crude calculation of dependency ratios – those of working age measured against those considered in retirement age. Within this framework 'independence' is so venerated that to be in need of care equates with being a burden on the diminishing resources.

Tronto (2013) rightly criticises the importation of care workers (women of colour who undertake the 'dirty work') as a 'rational' response to market requirements for cheaper and more available labour. Technological advances are also seen as a way of reducing the costs of care through limiting labour costs. In this construction technology replaces care. Notwithstanding the preferences of people who receive care, there are considerable problems, with the assumption of economic savings being the most important factor in the provision of care. This assumption misses the point: that care is difficult, situated, complex and requires in-depth understanding of care needs that cannot be achieved without interpersonal activities. Technologies may usefully complement care and should not be segregated by reference to 'cold technologies and warm care' (Pols and Moser, 2009) but, rather, integrated according to practices of care.

As Lloyd (2012) points out, the increase in numbers of older people has sharpened the 'moral message' within policy, making it clear that remaining healthy as we age is an individual responsibility and that those who fail to do so will be a drain on society. Aside from the lack of acknowledgement that older people are themselves care givers and major contributors to the care of others, the 'burden' discourse fuels arguments about intergenerational justice – pitting one generation against another and feeding ageism and negative attitudes towards older people and ageing. An ethic-of-care critique brings into view why the dominant framing of population ageing is so damaging:

> The value of an ethics of care perspective is that it does not differentiate between old (dependent) and young (independent) but sees dependency as inherent within the entire lifecourse and thus overcomes the tendency to regard older people as 'the other'. (Lloyd, 2012, p 4)

If we are to ensure that the ageing of the population is experienced positively at both an individual and a collective level, then the different ways of thinking offered by care ethics can help us towards this.

Book structure

This collection sets out the distinctiveness of a political ethic of care by reflecting on its challenge to dominant theoretical frameworks and practices of care, and its relationship to social justice and citizenship. To this end the collection includes the work of authors from the UK, Europe, North America, Africa and New Zealand working across different disciplinary fields including medicine and healthcare, social work, social policy, sociology, politics, psychology, international relations and geography. The key aims are:

- to reflect critically on the relationship between the growing interest in care ethics and current political and practice contexts
- to provide a timely contribution to theoretical developments and interest in care ethics

- to provide a resource for students, researchers and practitioners to know how to apply care-ethics analyses in their research or critiques of practice
- to bring together contributions from a diverse group of authors – established care ethicists, leaders in the field and new scholars
- to present previously unpublished theorisations that signpost future developments forming the basis of the next generation in the development of care ethics.

The chapters draw out and reflect upon the core themes discussed in this introductory chapter. The text is divided into two sections; the first explores theoretical and conceptual developments of an ethic of care, drawing on empirical material and policy and practice examples. This is based on a belief that a key strength of a care ethics framework is its relevance to applied contexts. In Chapter Two Joan Tronto argues for a global perspective on 'caring democracy'. Marian Barnes unpacks the significance of understanding caring relationships as constituting more than dyadic, intimate relationships in Chapter Three, while Lizzie Ward offers a critical perspective on the contemporary policy emphasis on 'self-care' in Chapter Four. Nicki Ward discusses how work on intersectionality and care ethics can usefully speak to each other in Chapter Five. The contribution from Amohia Boulton and Tula Brannelly in Chapter Six reflects the value of looking beyond dominant Western ways of thinking to explore Māori assumptions about the necessity of relationality rather than individuality for both well-being and justice. Vivienne Bozalek offers an innovative consideration of the operation of 'privileged irresponsibility' in the context of South Africa in Chapter Seven, while in Chapter Eight Diego de Merich engages in a critical dialogue between an ethic of justice and an ethic of care in the context of international development.

The contributions in the second section take more empirical work as their starting point. They consider how an ethic of care can be utilised to analyse and understand a range of subjective experiences in different geographical and cultural contexts. Ingunn Moser and Hilde Thygesen (Chapter Nine) explore how technology can contribute to a 'renewal' rather than be a 'replacement' for care, whilst Anne Liveng's perspective on Danish activity centres for older people highlights the tensions between logics of consumerism and care in Chapter Ten. The next two chapters consider how the AIDS/HIV epidemic has impacted on personal and power relationships in Sub-Saharan Africa. Anke Niehof argues in Chapter Eleven that we can see evidence of a matriarchy developing as a result of the significant roles taken on by women caring in this context. In Chapter Twelve Ruth Evans and Agnes Atim suggest that the involvement of people living with HIV can enhance 'relational autonomy' for both care givers and receivers, although this still reflects gendered roles. Nicki Ward in Chapter Thirteen and Ann Fudge Schormans in Chapter Fourteen also address issues of care, justice and recognition in relation to the position of people with learning disabilities, as care givers (Ward) and as expert critics on forms of visual representation (Fudge Schormans). Laura Steckley (Chapter Fifteen) addresses the challenging question of whether physical constraint can be considered a form of care. Teodora Manea (Chapter Sixteen) reminds us that 'care givers' – in this case doctors – can be in need of care and that migration can disrupt the support networks of those who might be regarded as powerful as well as those who are more obviously vulnerable. In Chapter Seventeen Brannelly returns us to the situation of those whose experience of 'care' is anything but caring and argues the necessity of bringing care and justice together in the treatment of people with mental illness.

In the conclusion we offer further reflections on the transformational potential of care ethics, based on the varied contributions to this book.

Note

[1] See Carers UK, www.carers.org/news/carers-save-uk-economy-%C2%A387-billion-year. http://www.carersuk.org/newsroom/item/2617-care-in-crisis-more-than-53-billion-wiped-from-the-economy.

TWO

Democratic caring and global care responsibilities

Joan Tronto

While feminist scholars long ago realised that care, and caring work, go beyond the household and are deeply implicated in national policies, the next great challenge is to transcend the national framework for care and to think about global responsibilities for care. That different states cope with the contemporary challenges of caring differently is obvious; indeed, a survey of these policies finds them to be 'worlds apart' (Razavi and Staab, 2012). But the concerns of care also *exceed* national boundaries, and the organising of care state by state presents further problems. In recent years, government policies throughout the globe have favoured solutions to the 'care deficit' that involve importing care labour from other countries (Yeates, 2004; Misra et al, 2006; Yea-huey, 2007; Benería, 2008; Boris and Parreñas, 2010; Elias, 2010; England and Henry, 2013). In welfare states, for example, a turn to individualised support has resulted in an increase in the in-migration of care workers. In other states, special provisions make it easier for employers to bring caring labourers across national borders. Such workers often find themselves unsupported as workers, and often abused. Relying upon them to solve the care problems of the advanced welfare states and other relatively richer sectors in other countries has the result of passing the 'care deficit' down the line and into other states. Passing the care deficit down the line makes it a less visible problem, and one that therefore attracts little serious political attention.

How and why might a democratic politics give priority to such issues?[1] In truth, if we take care as it is organised, and democracies as they exist, there is no solution to this problem. But if we think differently about care and democracy, and how it entails global responsibility, we might find a solution.

All humans need care every day of their lives; for some, their care needs are very well met, for others, their care needs go unmet. In general, those who receive more care are the ones who have the greatest resources; those with fewer resources receive less care (Hochschild,

2005). This imbalance is, as many have noted, a fundamental injustice. If we raise our concerns about care to the global level, the imbalance grows even greater. Ironically, those with the most pressing needs – hungry children in parts of the world where the risks of communicable disease are greatest – receive the least care. While it is true that the care policies of nation-states (with their diverse resources, commitments to public care, pressures for structural adjustment from international monetary and financial institutions, path-dependent historical circumstances, religious heritages and so forth) provide unevenly for care among their citizens, it is even more true when we look from a global level to see how these imbalances of care affect the lives of people around the globe (Heymann, 2006; WHO, 2009; Heymann and McNeill, 2012).

Other theorists of care have begun to think about what it would require to address global care imbalances. Fiona Robinson has written a powerful account of the need for greater cross-national care by arguing from the perspective of human security (Robinson, 2011). But before this critical engagement can effect genuine change, it requires that citizens in democracy accept the reasonableness of the human-security approach in the first place. Taking citizens as they are, this seems unlikely.

Virginia Held's (2008) account of her ethics of care treats the global as a meaningful level for care in addition to the level of the intimate interactions of the household. She writes that an ethics of care

> especially values caring relationships, obviously at the personal level within families and among friends and less obviously at the most general level of all human relationships.... It is appropriate for the wide but shallow human relations of global interactions, as well as for the strongest and most intimate human relations of care in families. (Held, 2008, pp 5–6)

Held allows that after the ethics of care, 'based on an experience that is universal – the experience of having been cared for, since no child can survive without this ...Then, it can conceptualize that within the more distant and weak relations of care, we can develop political and legal ways to interact' (Held, 2008, p 6), though she suggests that the ethics of care can also, at both the national and international levels, 'suggest alternative ways of interacting that may prove more satisfactory' than traditional institutions of justice:

These understandings can be matched at the international level, as care recommends respect for international law and also recommends alternative methods of fostering interconnection. We should work to build interactions that are not primarily political and legal – the often non-governmental networks of civil society, with their cultural, economic, educational, environmental, scientific, and social welfare forms of cooperative institution – and that will connect us and address our problems. We can gradually extend their reach so that we can better express our caring. (Held, 2008, p 7; footnote omitted)

On the one hand, Held's solution seems compelling; if non-governmental organisations can create connections that foster care, that is nothing but good. On the other hand, though, the problem that we are discussing here is already a problem of political and legal form, and one that, as national public policy, *obscures* the nature of the caring needs it is negatively affecting. Hoping that good will and civil society institutions can address this problem is too optimistic. Watching how caring crises increasingly affect the lives of migrants both at home and as they try to enter the US and Europe, it is clear that another approach to making care matter internationally needs to be tried.

As long as the nation-state remains the container within which care is allocated, then global unjust inequalities of care will exist. This is true, I shall argue here, not only because different nation-states have different ideas about their responsibilities to help out with caring for their citizens, but also because pushing care burdens to others (such as non-citizens) is a way to avoid the difficult questions about reallocating care within national contexts. An account of democratic caring requires a rethinking of the nature of responsibility itself. With such a rethinking, it might be possible to provide an account of caring in a global context that is not so unjust.

Organising care giving in an uncaring world order

The nation-state as container for care

Social welfare states vary tremendously in the generosity of the benefits they provide; numerous schemas to characterise social welfare systems distinguish them (Esping-Andersen, 1990). But in recent years, fuelled by the financial crises of the last decades, all social welfare states have increasingly arrived at two ways to 'contain' such costs. The first and obvious way to contain costs is to limit those who are eligible for benefits. Social welfare states have used a variety of means to achieve this end: introducing or tightening means tests, raising retirement ages, setting lifetime caps on healthcare reimbursements and so on. But this language of containment is actually useful to us in seeing some other dimensions of how states control costs. First, if we think of the container as impenetrable, then the state's control over its borders is a way to prevent the 'flood' of outsiders who might like to come to receive its generous provisions. In many countries in Europe, the Americas, Australia and wherever wealthier nations abut poorer ones, there is official or unofficial (illegal or vigilante) action to keep the outsiders out. On the other hand, second, the state also presents itself as a porous container when it allows undocumented workers to cross its borders to enter and provide care for citizens, especially without state sanction. The cost of such care is cheaper, the workers do not become a burden and the burden of care itself can be shifted back to private hands.

The fact that the nation-state has to appear to be a container that is both porous and impenetrable at once implies that something strange is going on. Indeed it is: the state can neither admit the seriousness of the needs for care without appearing inadequate nor admit the ways in which it has externalised the costs for caring by allowing the use of illegal workers. What it would take to fix such a problem is for states to face the real nature of the care deficit their increasingly vulnerable citizens face. Such a discussion is unlikely to happen under present circumstances.

The global market for care labour

Servants have laboured in the homes of those who are better off in most human societies, often doing the 'dirty work'. But contemporary forms of servantship are different: they are more global and more permanent, since servants now travel further from home. Servants in the past often served for only a part of their lives and then went on to do other things. As a result of this more permanent form for servantship, servants now are more likely to be marked by race, class and gender (Sarti, 2005; 2006). Numerous scholars have addressed the harms that come to individuals and their families, especially using the metaphor of the global care chain, a way to describe how the care deficit gets passed down the chain.

What is the significance of these changes? From a neoliberal economic standpoint, there is no problem; neoliberals argue that the individuals who enter the global care labour market are likely to be better off than if they had stayed at home (Bell, 2001). Remittances are a main form of revenue in the developing world today (Vila, 2004; Lutz, 2011; World Bank, 2013). Some scholars, for example Crozier, point to the 'significant benefits' to the 'well-being' of the families involved. Crozier goes further and observes benefits to societies as a whole of this transnational migration of caring labour: 'These benefits include the erosion of barriers to equality between genders and between households in wealthier and less wealthy nations' (Crozier, 2010, p 120). But Crozier's attempt to find a silver lining here ignores several factors. It is unclear that these barriers change much, especially as levels of economic inequality continue to widen. Further, the 'brain drain' of migration is another significant post-colonial justice problem (Buchan, 2001; Shachar, 2006; Asia Pulse Staff, 2009; Raghuram, 2009; Baputaki, 2009). Yet the problem is also serious when lower-status care workers leave their home countries. Such a 'care drain' is also a kind of 'brain drain'; to wit, the most ambitious, risk-taking people are leaving. When societies lose their 'best and brightest', they are harmed. Receiving nations receive concrete benefits from these migrant care exchanges without taking any responsibility for how they might affect the structures of sending societies (see Manea, Chapter Sixteen in this volume). While the question of responsibility can be avoided by assuming that global migration of care workers is only a question of individual action, realities belie that view. Some sending nations (such as the Philippines) actually encourage citizens to emigrate so as to provide foreign remittances (Parreñas, 2001). States are not simply bystanders in the global care market, they are active participants in how these markets operate.

Such involvement of the state is obscured by the belief that the standard for evaluation should be what individuals achieve for their well-being in the marketplace. Neoliberalism in itself is a great challenge for the provision of care. The mentality of the market is to suggest that the buying and selling of goods and services on the market will meet all needs. Thus, if a need is a real one, people will figure out how to use market forces to achieve their objective. If this means that those who are less well resourced end up with less-good care, then so be it. As market ideologies spread, the end result is to force each individual (or each family) back on its own devices to provide for its needed care.

Insecurity in the marketplace makes provision of care for oneself and loved ones precarious. In the face of such precarious circumstances, citizens demand that non-citizens should not 'take' resources that could be made available to them. This demand thus increases the incentive for the receiving states to appear as impermeable. At the same time, the economic dislocation and difficulties make it desirable for the sending states to perceive of the receiving states as permeable, and to some extent, they are, often through illegal migration.

These problems affect the provision of care itself; and the consequences are disastrous for the needy. But they are also disastrous for citizens in a democratic society. Democratic prospects narrow when citizens are encouraged to think about public life as only an extension of their own needs, and as not concerning the public weal (Wolin, 2008). When citizens have two different sets of standards to apply to the same phenomena depending upon whether or not they are the beneficiaries of the results, the problem is not only the violation of a formal rule of consistency. It also makes it more difficult for citizens to think in ethical terms at all, since they have already become hypocritical in some parts of their thinking.[2]

Are caring democracies the solution?

It is possible, however, to imagine and to articulate an alternative framework within which these questions might appear differently. This is as radical an idea as those proposed earlier from Robinson and Held. Nonetheless, I believe that the only way to proceed is first to 'uncontain' care within the nation-state, and then to move beyond the nation-state itself. This is not the same solution as simply ignoring the nation-state, but confronting and undoing its dual role of ignoring migrant care givers in order to make care provision easier, and vilifying them so as to assuage citizens' fears.

Caring democracy

While accounts of care differ in their breadth and depth, and while the concept is put to different uses in different contexts, I think it is fair to say that 'on the most general level', as Fisher and I put it in 1990, care is 'a species activity that includes everything that we do to maintain, continue and repair the world so that we may live in it as well as possible' (Fisher and Tronto, 1990, p 40). Almost all theorists who begin to speak about care in the context of the state immediately restrict care to an activity in which better-situated care givers help those who are in need (for example, Engster, 2007). Perhaps a better approach is to rethink this framework entirely.

Concepts are tools. It only makes sense, then, that as we move away from care 'on the most general level', to more specific forms of caring practices, the meaning of care will also shift with the more specific context. Yet concepts are not only tools, they also are always embedded in a context that is rich and full. Care's meaning will vary as well with the theoretical world-view within which it is placed. Caring has a different conceptual framework and justification in a society in which people's relationships are primarily feudal, or Confucian, or market-oriented. And caring has a different framework in a democratic society as well. What would a caring democracy, then, entail? (Tronto, 2013)

In the first instance, our understanding of democracy must change. Democracy is not simply giving people a voice. It is giving people a voice in the allocation of caring responsibilities. It also entails that all of those engaged in democratic political life must have the ability to voice their views on the proper allocation of caring responsibilities. Democracy understood in this way concerns the substance of democratic decisions, not just a procedure by which the people decide. Democracy needs to be focused on caring. If citizens decide, then, that they would like their democratic state to leave caring to the market, then they also need to take responsibility for that decision. Such an effort would force them to confront the questions: who is doing the caring in society? Do those individuals accept these responsibilities? Are they properly compensated for them?

Obviously, were such a genuine discussion of caring needs held, it would require that care deficits and care imbalances in society should be addressed. Other political values would come into different focus and require rethinking. Most importantly, equality needs reconceptualisation. In a caring democracy equality substantively involves the reality that all citizens are both agents and recipients of care. As a result, equality cannot be assumed to apply because everyone is predefined as an autonomous agent. Rather, the achievement of autonomy occurs out of a context within which one has been well cared for. Thus, vulnerability, rather than autonomy, is a better way to understand our basic equality.

The concept of caring also needs reworking. Fisher and Tronto (1990) defined caring as consisting of four phases: caring about, caring for, care giving and care receiving. Democratic caring requires a specifically democratic fifth phase of caring, 'caring with'. This fifth phase was presaged by the analysis offered by Selma Sevenhuijsen in *Citizenship and the Ethics of Care* (Sevenhuijsen, 1998). For Sevenhuijsen, public caring required importing two additional elements into the discussion of care: Habermasian-like discourse ethics, and a concept of trust.

Before turning to the fifth phase, consider how the other phases of care fit together. While in an integrated care process they would all fit together, the fifth phase builds expectations around tne 'feed-back loop' that works among the four phases. When care is responded to, through care receiving, and new needs are identified, individuals engaged in a care process return to the first phase and begin again. When, over time, people come to expect that there will be such ongoing engagements in care processes with others, then we have arrived at caring with. The virtues of such caring with are trust and solidarity. Trust builds as people realise that they can rely upon others to participate in their care and care activities. Solidarity forms when citizens come to understand that they are better off engaged in such processes of care together, rather than alone.

How would caring democracies approach the problems of care deficits? Surely it would not be acceptable to pass them along to the most vulnerable. Nor would allowing the importation of care labour to solve care deficits work. From this perspective the hypocrisy of allowing care workers to enter the state in order to provide care work takes on a different meaning.

Caring democracies and nation-states as containers of care

Making care democratic on a global level is a tall order. But if the approach suggested here is correct, then it requires even more conceptual change. Not only do the relationships among the nation-state 'containers' need to change, but change is necessary within them as well. As Christine Koggel has noted, change cannot be left only to others (Koggel, 2006; 2008; 2009).

There are some clear directions that a genuinely caring democracy might want to take. The first is to follow a 'modest proposal' that has been made to extend citizenship to anyone who is involved in a relationship of care with a citizen (Tronto, 2005, and see, for example Crozier (2010). If we start from the premise of caring democracy as an allocation of caring responsibilities, then it obviously follows that the caring responsibilities of those who are doing care work within any society have to be included within this discussion. This proposal is more radical than other current proposals about providing amnesties for workers already in a country that is using their care labour. It is probably too radical to be implemented, but it forces people to confront directly the questions about how they are taking advantage of the labour of migrants.

While no one actually lives yet in caring democracies, it is difficult to imagine that 'caring with' migrant workers will evoke sufficient reflection to correct the harms that are done to them. Since this is the case, what else can be done?

Two obvious steps suggest themselves:

First, people can work in solidarity with global care workers. Domestics are increasingly well organised and politically powerful everywhere. In recent years, the International Labour Organisation adopted Convention 189, which entered into force in September 2013. The Convention provides basic rights for workers in domestic settings. Within nation-states, some labour laws now protect workers; New York State has extended worker protection, overtime hours and so forth, to those who work in domestic settings. Global care workers have organised themselves into the International Domestic Workers' Network in October 2013 (International Labour Organisation, 2013).

Second, and more broadly, we can articulate an alternative vision to the neoliberal order. The insight of Ghassan Hage here is key:

> The global/transcendental corporation needs the state, but does not need the nation. National and sub-national (such as state or provincial) governments all over the world are transformed from being primarily the managers of a national society to being the managers of the aesthetics of investment space. Among the many questions that guide government policy, one becomes increasingly paramount: how are we to make ourselves *attractive* enough to entice this transcendental capital hovering above us to land in our nation? (Hage, 2003, p 19)

Caring does not need the nation, either. Indeed, a nation that defines itself in terms of the groups who are properly citizens is likely to exploit others as foreign care workers. Caring needs the state, but a state that is sensitive to the needs of its citizens and not just to the needs of the corporations who might someday pass down economic advantages to citizens. And caring needs a state that is radically democratic in thinking through whom and how to meet those caring needs.

Conclusion

A very different kind of democratic politics will be necessary to notice the moral harm currently done in a system of caring that at best protects care givers and receivers who happen to be national citizens. Calling current states on their hypocritical willingness to contain care both tightly and loosely may begin to move our ways of thinking about these matters. To do so, though, requires us to change profoundly how we think about democracy by putting care and its complex responsibilities at democracy's core.

Notes

[1] I am deeply indebted to Marian Barnes, who initially posed this question to me in this way, and to the participants of the conference whose comments helped me to clarify my views.

[2] I take this important point, that one should never overlook the importance of making citizens act hypocritically, from Claudia Card's objection to ROTC (Reserve Officer Training Corps) on campus during the era of 'don't ask/don't tell' policies for gays and lesbians in the military. See C. Card (1995) *Lesbian Choices,* New York: Columbia University Press.

THREE

Beyond the dyad: exploring the multidimensionality of care

Marian Barnes

Introduction

This collection of essays, and much recent work on the ethics of care, has sought to expand our understanding of care in terms of its transformative potential in both political and personal contexts. As is so often the case, it is the work of Joan Tronto that points us in this direction. Joan Tronto and Berenice Fisher define care as follows:

> On the most general level, we suggest that caring be viewed as a species activity that includes everything that we do to maintain, continue, and repair our 'world' so that we can live in it as well as possible. That world includes our bodies, our selves, and our environment, all of which we seek to interweave in a complex, life-sustaining web. (Quoted in Tronto, 1993, p 103)

This definition asks us to consider the significance of care in the multiplicity of ways in which we seek to look after and improve ('repair') our interpersonal, social and physical environment. It names care as a necessity for us all, and it recognises that it is interdependence, not independence, that characterises the human condition. It is a way of thinking about care that has made possible critical scholarship and empirical work that applies new ethical perspectives on issues such as domestic violence (Held, 2010) and international relations (Robinson, 1999), as well as on the intimate personal relationships more usually considered as the domain of care.

But we continue to have a problem. The word 'care' is a loaded one and resistances to its use as well as scepticism about its value suggest that we need to be prepared to offer up more precise ways of understanding what we mean by care when we advocate the value of care thinking in different contexts. In this chapter I offer some pointers towards diversifying our understanding of what care is, what motivates and sustains care in different contexts and what this implies for an ethic of care that enhances social justice.

Origins

Much early work on care ethics (in particular that of Noddings, 1984) took the mother–child relationship as the quintessential care relationship. Noddings recognised the relationality of caring. She understood this in terms of how the cared-for person receives care, that this is a necessary part of care and thus that the ethics of care includes experiences of and responses to 'being cared for' (Noddings, 1996a, p 35). But she understands care as a 'particular type of relationship between two people' (Noddings, 1996b, p 160) and her work on care within education is framed within this perspective. This focus on mothering as the archetype of care has had the consequence of understanding care as a private relationship between two individuals, one of whom occupies a powerful position *vis-à-vis* the other. Images of mothers and their babies, whether artistic representations of the Madonna and child or advertising images intended to sell baby milk products, focus on the entwined pair, an intimate relationship from which others are excluded. They often seem disconnected from other people and the world outside, contained within their own space and time. The baby is utterly dependent on her mother to support her. The mother is tender, but powerful in response to this vulnerability.

The power of this (common sense) understanding of the source of care within the mother–child relationship is reflected in Hollway's (2006) exploration of 'the capacity to care'. Although Hollway seeks to expand her analysis to 'explore how the capacity to care is implicated in institutional change and caring about strangers across difference and distance' (p 2), her starting point is in maternal care and the way in which caring capacity develops through interactions between mothers and their male and female children. While we are all, as Kittay (1999) reminds us, 'some mother's child' and thus know, in some way, of the necessity of care, we are not all mothers and thus cannot all develop our capacity to care through the practice of caring for a vulnerable infant. Understanding what care is on the basis of the particular relationship between mother and child, comprising a particular type of vulnerability, powerlessness, intensity and exclusiveness, can be seen as a problematic starting point for understanding care in the much broader way that a critical and political ethic of care offers.

Developments

A position that emphasises inequality, vulnerability and uni-directionality within caring relationships underpins the rejection of 'care' per se by many of those identified as occupying the 'needy' position within a care dyad. And yet recognition of vulnerability, and both political and personal responsibility to attend to and take action to meet needs associated with vulnerability, underpin arguments for care as both an ethical and a political necessity. As work on the ethics of care has developed we can see how various strands of thinking have sought to deal with this. Firstly, recent work that explores care within the context of interpersonal relationships has sought to develop the potential within care ethics to recognise care as a two-way practice in which the contribution of the 'care receiver' to the process of care is essential to the completion of care (for example, Pettersen and Hem, 2011). Empirical studies have also highlighted the cultural significance of reciprocity and its potential role in facilitating care receiving when people are reluctant to admit to a need for care (Ward, L. et al, 2012). In my recent work I have sought to expand on the importance of understanding reciprocity within care without assuming a contractual basis for this (Barnes, 2012a).

There is also increasing recognition that the identities of 'care giver' and 'care receiver' are fluid and dynamic (Ward, N., 2011 and Chapter Five in this volume); that care can be and is given and received among groups, including those who may be defined by their need to receive care (Emond, 2003); that it is often the case that there is more than one care giver in any caring relationship (Kittay, 1999), and that even when the care relationship may consist primarily of two people, then the capacity of the carer to continue to care is dependent on support offered to her by others – Kittay's 'nested dependencies'. It is also the case that people's caring histories mean that they are involved in different caring relationships throughout their lifetime, not only moving between identities as care givers and care receivers, but also experiencing what care means in very different ways as they seek to care for, for example, a son with mental health problems and a spouse with dementia, or as they take part in collective action with others experiencing stigmatisation or marginalisation (Barnes, 2006).

Finally, there is the now significant body of work that addresses the issue of care without assuming interpersonal relationships between individuals known to each other. This includes Robinson's (1999) work on care as a value in international relations and other work that considers care in a global context (for example, Pulcini, 2009;

Scuzzarello et al, 2009). This all reinforces the inadequacy of basing our understanding of what care *is* on what we all think we know about relations between mothers and infants. The disciplinary diversity of work on care in a multiplicity of contexts – from philosophy to psychology and politics as well as applied disciplines such as social policy, nursing and gender studies, contributes to the different ways in which the concept of care is employed, and arguably adds to the difficulty of trying to develop a framework within which we can talk to each other about what care is in different contexts. Nevertheless, we need to attempt some summary of where work on the ethics of care has got to in terms of what care means. My starting point is located in my perspective as an applied social scientist with a commitment to understanding the lived experience of those involved in caring relationships, but also to the necessity of critical analysis reflecting both the moral and political character of care. The capacity of care ethics to engage with both perspectives is what gives it its force. Tronto's identification of care as necessary to 'repair[ing] our world' and Sevenhuijsen's (2004) inclusion of 'renewal' in her framework for policy analysis that goes beyond a critical discourse analysis and into an exploration of how things could be different identify the ethics of care as fundamentally concerned with making change. That is a perspective that informs this collection as a whole.

It is clear that it is inadequate to understand the care relationship solely as dyadic, or to identify one type of relationship as defining care. If we are to accept that it is useful to think of care as a 'species activity' and one that encompasses relationships that are not only intimate, or interpersonal, but also political and stretching across boundaries that distinguish and separate those who recognise membership of some shared polis, identity or both, then we need to attempt some way of capturing both the similarities and differences in what we mean by care.

My aim here is not to suggest a series of categorical distinctions that constrain creativity or imagination about care. One of the key insights and foundational perspectives of care ethics is the necessity for deliberation in response to the specific contexts in which need is experienced, and the inadequacy of abstract principles to practices to enable social justice. I thus offer this analysis as a heuristic device to encourage dialogue, rather than as a system of classification or listing of variables against which to measure care. As will become evident, the different characteristics of care that I consider below are interconnected – and while I consider each separately, it is how they interact with each other that constitutes the meaning of care in any particular situation, and the specific ethical issues associated with this. My argument here reflects Tronto's articulation of the dimensions of care that together constitute care's integrity (1993, p 136).

Networks and collectives

I start with one of the most practical ways in which we need to understand care beyond dyadic relationships – by recognising the significance of the broader sets of relationships within which relationships between those identified as care givers and care receivers are embedded. This is not to ignore the common experience of those who identify themselves or may be identified as 'carers' of being left alone to shoulder a substantial task of caring for a disabled child, elderly partner or parent. Rather, it is to recognise that a political ethics of care that understands individuals as relational subjects existing within networks of ties and reciprocal connections would consider such isolation as a failure of the shared responsibility to care. There is much empirical evidence about the importance of support networks and the damaging impact of isolation experienced by those who are 'sole carers' that supports this. And at an interpersonal level within families the explicit or implicit negotiations that take place about who will care can be understood to reflect the working out of moral obligations embodying lay ethics in practice (Finch and Mason, 1993). Thus we need to explore the different ways in which shared responsibilities for care can and should be enabled to happen.

In order to do this I suggest that we need to distinguish what might be called 'networked care': care that is given and received within networks that may include both paid and unpaid care givers (family members, friends and care workers), who may or may not live together or even encounter each other on a regular basis; and 'collective care', by which I mean care that is often reciprocal, that emerges through frequent interactions among groups of people who often share similar characteristics or circumstances (as in the case of residential living, or among user groups engaged in collective action for transformative change, Barnes 2007).

What I am calling 'networked care' reflects aspects of Kittay's (1999, p 67) arguments about 'nested dependencies' or 'nested obligations'. If giving care is not to impact adversely on the carer's well-being, then she should be entitled to support in her own right. But this should not solely depend on unpaid input from family and friends; rather, it is a responsibility of states. One of the aims of an information and support programme for carers of people with dementia was to encourage carers to identify their support network and to recognise its importance. One of the negative emotional impacts of the programme was experienced by carers unable to identify such a network and for whom the time-limited nature of the programme was a disappointment because it did not create an enduring network (Barnes et al, 2014). 'Care for the carers' has been a campaign slogan from the early days of the UK Carers Movement. Kittay (1999, p 133) identifies the principle of *doulia* – a concept of social cooperation deriving from the Greek word for service – as providing the basis for social welfare in which there is collective responsibility to look after the well-being of those providing hands-on care within the private sphere. In some welfare states this has led to policy and practice initiatives encouraging carers to identify themselves as such, and offering practical and emotional support that is designed both to minimise adverse impacts of care giving and to encourage a continued capacity and willingness to care so as to prevent additional demands on the state.

But these dual objectives highlight the importance of the critical policy analysis from an ethic of care that Sevenhuijsen (1998) has promoted and undertaken and that others have taken up (for example, Barnes, 2011; Williams, 2004b). Policies that derive from an essentialised view of the superiority of family care and a concept of responsibility that locates this within private lives and not within collective responsibilities, including those of states to ensure well-being and justice, do not fulfil the requirements of what Tronto describes as a democratic and caring society 'whose account of justice balances how the burdens and joys of caring are equalized so as to leave every citizen with as much freedom as possible' (Tronto, 2013, p 46). Kittay (1999) recognises her privileged position in being able to both identify and pay for someone with whom she can share the care of her daughter in a way that she describes as 'distributed mothering' (p 156). Such private arrangements can emerge out of family and friendship networks as well as via the market. But if *doulia* is to be both democratic and detached from obligations linked to the preventative imperatives of social policy, then state support is essential.

A key implication of recognising the significance of caring networks is that responsibilities for and to care need to be understood to operate within the network as a whole, rather than being solely in one direction – from care giver to care receiver. Responsibilities exist to other members of the network and attentiveness to the range of others contributes to the complexity of caring relationships. This in turn emphasises the importance of both dialogue and praxis to enable the learning that is necessary for ethical care. Interdependency is multidirectional.

What I am calling 'collective care' offers a rather different perspective on the way in which care is generated through interactions involving a number of people. While caring networks can be understood to focus on the needs of an individual (a disabled child, a parent with dementia, for example) and the shared responsibilities for meeting those needs, collective care emerges out of interactions between individuals who share similar needs by virtue of their circumstances, such as young people in residential care, or identities, for example people with mental health problems working together in an advocacy organisation. What characterises these contexts is the greater equality between those who 'care for' and those who receive care in what are often reciprocal relationships. This does not mean an absence of conflict, nor that there may be times when care is given and received in a particular direction. But evidence of the importance of collective relationships, in particular among those often constructed as care receivers, unsettles assumptions about vulnerabilities residing within individuals rather than produced within relational contexts (Emond, 2012).

Such contexts also suggest a rather different view of responsibility to care. Even in the socio-cultural construction of responsibility adopted by care ethicists there is an assumption of some link between responsibility and unequal power – because of the dominance of a view of care as a relationship between an individual in need and another (or others) with the capability to meet that need. How, then, should we understand the responsibilities of those with equal or similar needs? Perhaps the answer requires us to recognise another insight of care ethics, which is that the need to care and the importance of caring for are also shared. We all need to recognise not only our vulnerability, but also that being able to care for others is both a right and a source of satisfaction (Lynch et al, 2009). Recognising the contribution made to the care of others by those identified as 'problems' (such as young people in residential care, Emond, 2012) or as in need of care (such as people with learning difficulties, see N. Ward and Fudge Schormans, Chapters Thirteen and Fourteen in this volume) not only unsettles the care giver–care receiver dichotomy, but also asks us to value spaces where collective living or other forms of collaboration can generate and support care.

An understanding of caring networks and of collective care emphasises both the relational and social characteristics of care and the inadequacy of a focus on individual subjects detached from personal and social networks.

Presence/distance

The archetype of the caring relationship is a face-to-face relationship in which the care giver is not only physically present for the care receiver, but also emotionally present and focused on the other to whom care is given. Caring involves both physical touch and bodily tending as well as an attentiveness to the needs that give rise to this and the responses it evokes. But caring also involves organisational labour, and caring networks imply that activity on behalf of the other done at a distance, and the support offered to the hands-on care giver, should be understood as constituting care. Thus physical presence is not always necessary for care.

However, attentiveness to the particularity of the circumstance of the person in need of care, the importance of recognising responses to care and the circumstances giving rise to the need for this, and the dialogic practices necessary to enable care, mean that, if all those involved in caring networks are not present, the imperative to create spaces for dialogue between them is great. In practical terms practices that recognise 'care work' only as taking place when a worker is in the home of a service user, that relegate office space to the cars that workers use to travel from one service user to another and that understand professional supervision as performance monitoring rather than a space for discussion about ethical and practice dilemmas, deny the shared dialogic space necessary for effective care.

But we also need to consider how those responsible for making policies for care, but whose jobs do not require them to come into direct contact with care receivers, can develop and practise the attentiveness necessary to create the policy and institutional contexts necessary for care. In Barnes (2008) I discuss one aspect of this in exploring 'care full deliberation' between officials and service users. Mackay (2001) considers the impact on political processes and on decision making of the presence within political forums of those with acknowledged experience of care. The general point here is that a political ethic of care necessitates articulating the responsibility of those who do not come into the presence of care receivers in the context of hands-on care giving to act and deliberate carefully. That is, that care thinking and moral imagination are necessary regardless of physical presence, and that the presence of caring practices within policy processes is necessary to the 'caring democracy' that Tronto (2013) calls for.

That care for unknown others is both necessary and possible has been argued by those adopting a global perspective on justice (for example, Robinson, 1999). Closer to home, work on information and communications technology is exploring the impact of electronic media in enabling the development of caring relationships among those who may never come into face-to-face contact. Both bodies of work demonstrate that we cannot understand care as solely generated and practised through relationships involving physical presence, but that what care *is* will change in respect to this and attention is needed to how it is and can be generated in such contexts. To care for unknown others demands a moral imagination that transcends the immediate and concrete stimulus of interpersonal interaction or the recognition of apparent shared interests promoted by communitarian values. It is prompted by recognition of the vulnerability of us all and by an acceptance of responsibility that goes beyond that felt for those within our inner circle. A major contribution of work on the ethics of care in this context is to understand that interdependence is not restricted to interpersonal networks, but extends through interactions with those we may come into contact with on a temporary basis at times of specific need (personal crisis or a broader catastrophe with collective impact), and to those distant from us both spatially and culturally, but with whom we share occupancy of the globe.

Intimacy

Related to the above is the third dimension we need to understand as contributing to the diversity of care: that is, the degree of intimacy involved. The archetype I started with – that of the mother and child – is defined both by physical presence and emotional intimacy. Similarly, spouse/partner relationships and, to a lesser but nevertheless significant extent, caring relationships between adult children and their parents or between siblings or other family members both benefit from and are constrained by emotional connections and socially constructed assumptions about duty and power (Barnes, 2006 and 2012b). These motivating factors are different from, but interact with, those driving professional or other paid care giving.

Engster (2007) sets out a hierarchy of caring obligations based in the degree of intimacy and physical connection between those in need and those giving care. His first level of responsibility is care for self (see Ward, L., Chapter Four in this volume) arguing that unless we care for ourselves we will not be in a position to care for others. But it is not only in the assumed and/or accepted degree of responsibility experienced that we need to consider differences in care and intimacy. Care giving and receiving is tied up with identity and subjectivity forged though different types of relationship. How we respond to care depends not only on how it is given but on who gives it. It is not necessarily the case that care receivers prefer care to be given within existing intimate relationships – for example, some disabled people have spoken of the negative impact of intimate care on sexual relationships between partners, while for others the intimate tending that comprises much physical care is experienced as an act of love.

Once again, the insight of care ethics is to focus our attention on the particularity of the specific relational context for care and to name as a moral as well as interpersonal issue the question of how we practise in response to this.

Time

Finally, we need to understand both the personal and political issues associated with recognising the temporal dimension of care. The practice of care takes place through time and Tronto's characterisation of the 'phases' of care suggests not only that being attentive and caring about are precursors to actions involved in arranging or giving hands-on care, but that what constitutes the work of care will shift in response both to changing needs and to the internal dynamics of the caring relationship. Thus, while intimate care giving and receiving is experienced in the present, and that present can appear to occupy the whole of time for those who can feel trapped within the immediacy and constancy of needs to be met, care has its own trajectory that encompasses not only the present but the individual and shared histories of those involved in caring relationships, and anxiety, fear, anticipation or hope about the future. The stories told to me by family carers (Barnes, 2006) revealed the impact of past relationships and experiences on current care: including the challenges associated with caring for a husband who became ill at the point at which the marriage was breaking down, and the impact of a history of alcoholism and marital conflict on a son's preparedness to care for his mother. But these stories also highlighted the significance of perceived futures – whether those were fears that a severely disabled child would not survive, concern about what would happen following the death of a carer, or optimism that disability would not be a barrier to quality of life. The varied capacity of care givers to encompass understanding of likely future scenarios within the immediacy of their current caring relationships was evident in research into the responses of carers of people with dementia to information designed to enable them to care better for their relative (Barnes and Henwood, 2015). It appeared that the capacity to care over time was not always enhanced by knowing more about what that future might involve.

The importance of recognising the significance of the temporal dimension of caring relationships is positively reflected in the use of life-history books with children who have entered the 'looked after' system and who may experience a range of different placements with different carers. The absence of such recognition can be a source of frustration when paid workers evidence no interest in what people were like before their frailties led to intervention. Professional care relationships start at the point of need and end when this is no longer assessed as entitling support, whereas personal ones are embedded in previous relationships and are defined not solely by need. And yet, unlike 'treatment' that is predicated on an assumption that its application will obviate the need that gave rise to it, care has no end point. People do not 'stop caring', unless some fracture too great to overcome intervenes. Neither admission to a nursing home nor death (McCarthy, 2013) marks the end of care.

The impact of past injustice may be implicated in both the need for and capacity to receive care. The rejection of care often has its origins in experiences of professionalised services as paternalistic, oppressive and sometimes abusive, and of family care as protective if not smothering. As Boulton and Brannelly (Chapter Six in this volume) highlight, past injustices resulting in discrimination, inequality and poverty challenge us to take responsibility not only to recognise how past injustice affects present behaviour, but also for ensuring the conditions in which amelioration can be achieved. In addition to the enduring injustices wrought by colonisation, other traumas resulting from the holocaust, from ethnic cleansing and apartheid (Bozalek, Chapter Seven in this volume) raise ethical, political and practical questions about collective responsibilities that cannot adequately be answered by an appeal solely to justice. As Pulcini (2009) argues, care goes beyond the repairing of wrongs and asserting impartial principles of equity; care also aims to 'affirm and repeat the *value of the bond*' (p 250, emphasis in original) and thus to break the cycle of injustice and redress. Whatever its flaws, we can see attempts to put this into practice in the Truth and Reconciliation Commission in post-apartheid South Africa.

Time also defines one aspect of the presence/distance dimension of care. Future generations are not immediately present to us, but will be affected by decisions made now. Care requires responsibility for the future. The significance of this includes the way in which we make policies for older people. The national insurance system in the UK embodied notions of collective responsibility to older people and also to those who may find themselves unable to work. What has been called the 'intergenerational contract' (Walker, 1996) reflects a commitment to responsibilities to maintain and support the bond between generations. Contemporary attempts to whip up conflict between younger and older people unsettle the notion that not only should we care for those who are currently old, but also we should care about our future selves. Broader cultural and popular discourses that name old age as something to be personally resisted and even 'prevented' shut us off from attentiveness to the experience of old age and from the responsibility to enable positive relationships between old and young.

Implicated in such responses is the fear of what it means to be old and this, in turn, is associated with fear about both abandonment and abuse within what is meant to be the 'care system'. But awareness of our personal vulnerability that may increase as we age sits alongside awareness of our collective vulnerability in the face of a failure to care about the world we will leave for future generations. Pulcini (2009) links fear to the potential for awakening the imagination necessary to anticipate the consequences of a failure to act to repair our physical as well as social world. Neither compassion, she argues, nor indignation is enough to mobilise us in this way. Rather, this requires 'the awareness, which can only belong to a relational subject, that we are part of a common and vulnerable humankind, of a generational chain that binds us to the fate of future generations' (p 251).

Conclusion

In this chapter I have to sought to summarise the multiple dimensions of care that mean we cannot understand this solely as a relationship between two people. I am not suggesting that we should develop a categorisation of different 'types' of care, but rather that we should be attentive to the way in which these intersect and constitute the complexity and diversity of care. Tronto's work and that which has followed has deliberately sought to expand our conception of what care is. This has been a vital part of the project to recognise care as political as well as personal and to locate us all within care. But some have been uneasy about the inclusiveness of the Tronto and Fisher definition and developments within the ethics of care literature now enable us to expand upon the implications of such a broad conception of care. This enables us to recognise the varied origins of and motivations for care at both personal and political levels. It reinforces the importance of deliberation not only among those directly involved in caring relationships, but also involving those whose actions shape the discursive and policy contexts within which care happens. Developing the capacity to care requires developing imagination that can reach out to unknown others across both space and time. Such dialogue must include the different voices of those for whom care is an acknowledged imperative in their everyday lives, and whose current experiences are marred by histories of colonisation, oppression and discrimination. Care full deliberation, capable of stimulating the necessary moral imagination, requires encompassing 'emotional morality' (Barnes, 2008). A caring democracy requires new forms of caring practices within decision making as well as within face-to-face care giving and receiving. It is via these routes that care can achieve the transformations that justice claims alone cannot.

FOUR

Caring for ourselves?
Self-care and neoliberalism

Lizzie Ward

Introduction

Caring for 'ourselves' forms part of the broad definition of care outlined by Tronto and Fisher as one aspect of 'everything we do to maintain, continue and repair our world' (Tronto, 1993). But thinking about what exactly 'self-care' means and the ways in which it has been interpreted and mobilised in different contexts tells us that this is a term with multiple and contested meanings. Over recent years the concept of 'self-care' has been mobilised by policy makers and governments in the deepening of neoliberal objectives to dismantle public welfare resources and shift responsibility for care onto individual citizens. Yet ideas about self-care have a longer and wider history as part of collective struggles – for recognition of the experiences of disabled people, of women's health movements challenging medical hierarchies and in contexts of community-led peer support and self-help groups. This chapter examines the origins and contexts of self-care and how it is currently deployed in neoliberal restructuring of welfare systems. I illustrate this by specific reference to UK health and welfare policies and interventions to offer an analysis, grounded in care ethics, of the wider political implications for responsibilities for care in the dismantling of welfare states.

In advanced capitalist welfare states, such as the UK, the restructuring that has been underway since the late 1970s has eroded the conditions of the post-war social contract between states and citizens. Over time, part of this process has been to change people's expectations about the respective responsibilities of state and citizen. More recently and under the cloak of austerity measures and financial crises, the justification for further cuts to welfare and health budgets has been framed, at least in the UK, through the repeated articulation of discourses that present immutable 'facts' as to why the reforms are necessary. Firstly, that public-funded welfare systems are unsustainable and we simply cannot afford them as health and social care needs increase; secondly that welfare systems that are too 'generous' create dependency, and thus stifle innovation and creativity; thirdly, that individual 'choice' is paramount and freeing people from paternalistic welfare will lead to individual 'empowerment'.

Self-care has increasingly been used in health and care policies in this context, often presented as a logical response to demographic change, particularly population ageing, and the anticipated increased demand on health and care resources. Within the UK, self-care has been mobilised in policy initiatives in the self-management of long-term health conditions and through health promotion in relation to diet, exercise, smoking and alcohol consumption. It includes targeting specific population groups (such as people who live in areas of economic deprivation as well as people over the age of 50), to take responsibility for their own health and well-being through promoting changes in individual behaviour and life-style.

Self-care from the perspective of care ethics

As a concept, 'self-care' is a valuable ideological tool not only because it appeals to common-sense notions of individual empowerment and greater choice and control, but more significantly because it fits neoliberal economic imperatives to place responsibilities for health and welfare firmly with individual citizens. By constructing care as an individual responsibility of the 'self', the normative policy framework that has emerged furthers existing inequalities by obscuring the collective responsibility of the state to provide adequately for its citizens. Care ethics, in contrast, highlights the fundamental place of care to human life and thus the political implications that follow from this, including the responsibilities of governments for ensuring care.

Care ethics has provided a robust critique of liberal autonomy and its failure to capture the messy interdependencies of lived lives by assuming 'each citizen to be a detached individual, whose aim is autonomous behaviour, who needs nobody and who recognises dependency and vulnerability in others' (Sevenhuijsen 1998, p 28). In addition to failing to recognise the universality of human care needs the neoliberal paradigm is thus harmful in the way that it 'objectifies otherness' and encourages the idea that needs and dependency feature only in others' lives and not our own (Tronto, 1993; Sevenhuijsen, 1998; Kittay, 1999). In reality we do not divide neatly into 'care givers' and 'care receivers' – we are all implicated. Those who give care also have care needs, those who receive care can be givers (see Ward, N., Chapter Thirteen in this volume). Acknowledging care needs in one's 'self' may dislodge the 'othering' and rupture the binary division between care giving and receiving.

Within an ethics of care framework self and autonomy are conceptualised as relational, that is, a self embedded in relationships with others who attains autonomy through relationships. Care needs are met through relationships between people and within networks of people. This includes the ways in which we meet our own self-care needs, which, like all other aspects of care, are relational. Rather than the individualised notion that dominates policy discourses, self-care may be better understood as part of 'collective care' and/or 'networked care' (see Barnes, Chapter Three in this volume).

In rejecting autonomy as an abstract concept, care ethics calls attention to the everyday lived experiences of care practices. Learning from, and paying attention to, the experiences and knowledge of care receivers is the epistemological dimension that is central in care ethics. This is not only vital for understanding care in practice through the element of 'responsiveness' at an individual level; the collective experiences of care receivers and givers have been instrumental in the emergence of self-help and user groups. As the next section shows, it is precisely because the lived experiences of service users have not been listened to by professionals that ideas around self-help and self-care have evolved.

Self-help to self-care: from collective struggle to neoliberal co-option

The emergence of self-help campaigns and initiatives on health and welfare has been linked to the political and social movements of the 1960s and 1970s. This period has been characterised by challenges to traditional forms of authority through the emergence of a 'counter-culture' producing alternative ways and means of understanding the world. Among these, feminist health campaigns were at the forefront of collective struggles to challenge the power of medicalised knowledge of women's bodies in relation to areas of healthcare such as childbirth, contraception and reproduction. At the core of these campaigns was the notion of 'self-help' and women coming together in groups to share experience and knowledge. The 1978 British edition of *Our Bodies Ourselves* charts the growth of these groups and is illustrative of the '*by* women *for* women' approach to increase women's own self-knowledge of their bodies and as a way of gaining a sense of control over their lives and health. This, however, was not simply about personal empowerment or an individual pursuit but, rather, it was inseparable from the collective struggle to achieve social change and adequate health and care resources from the state. Considered a classic women's liberation text, *Our Bodies Ourselves*, itself the result of women's coming together through the Boston Women's Health Book Collective, provided something of a blueprint to encourage other women to form self-help groups:

> Self-help is a political act. It is deeply challenging to the existing health care system. Through sharing our knowledge collectively we have developed skills – we, not only the 'professionals', will know what is done to us medically but why it is done. We do not take the place of the doctor, but we do reverse the patriarchal-authority-doctor-over-'patient' roles. (Phillips and Rakusen, 1978, p 561)

Collective ways of organising for mutual support can also be found in self-help groups that have grown out of a lack of recognition of the knowledge and experiences of people living with a health condition or impairment. Kendall and Rogers have termed this a 're-appropriation of medicine by lay people' (Kendall and Rogers, 2007, p 131), in which values such as mutual support based on a shared collective identity challenge the power of health professionals to marginalise the experiences of people who use services. Self-help groups, they argue, offer 'mutual support and friendship; fundraising for research; information and learning resources; a safe haven for people with stigmatized conditions and a lobby for recognition and support'. It is shared identities and experiences of marginalisation that are important here in resisting medicalised knowledge and challenge 'the health professional monopoly and the political assumptions of corporate rationalization' (Kendall and Rogers, 2007, p 132).

Under the umbrella term of self-help groups that have developed within the UK we could include groups of people who come together on the basis of a specific health condition; people who use mental health services; people who identify with a broader disability movement; as well as carers and locally based community support groups. While there is enormous diversity in the range of ways in which these groups operate, in their size and scale and their different objectives, they demonstrate different ways of offering support among people who share experiences of marginalisation (Barnes, 2007). Overall, they have contributed to a collective challenge to the knowledge and expertise of health and social care professionals. The demand to be heard as experts in their own lives, and for the right to be involved in decisions about service provision, treatment, care and in research, has impacted widely within the health and social care system since the mid-1990s. That is not to suggest, however, that this has been a straightforward process, but, rather, one that is fraught with political struggles over power and meaning. Inevitably perhaps, as the need to include service users' 'voice' has become more accepted into the mainstream, the 'voice' has become less radical and more open to different interpretations.

Most significantly, what might be understood as progressive social change, 'patient empowerment' or greater control for service users, has taken place within the context of the restructuring of the health and welfare systems, increased privatisation and the organisation of public resources on market principles. The danger of co-option therefore has always been part of the political engagement between user groups and professionals and policy makers. The arguments of those campaigning for change have been most successful when they have found accommodation within the dominant political agendas. Reflecting on the success of the disability movement's campaign to secure direct payments (for care services), Jenny Morris notes:

> The resulting legislation, passed by a Conservative government in 1996, fitted in with an agenda which sought the privatisation of services and an undermining of public sector trade unions. While disabled people's organisations did not support such policies, we did − when making the case for direct payments − use language which fitted well with the individualist political framework which was becoming more and more dominant. Thus we emphasised disabled people's rights to autonomy and self-determination, which resonated with the Conservative Government's agenda; and drew attention to the way a lack of choice and control could undermine human rights, which then fitted well with New Labour's agenda. (Morris, 2011, p 3)

The emphasis on personal responsibility and self-reliance has been a dominant feature of UK political agendas since the Thatcherite period in the 1980s. The (continual) restructuring of both the National Health Service (NHS) and welfare system, under the guise of efficiency, through the introduction of competition and contracting-out of services to the private sector has become something of a permanent feature since then. Although the tone and language have varied through successive governments, the direction of travel has been constant, as has been the appeal to consumerist notions of 'choice'.

Bella (2010) argues that public health and health promotion have become reconfigured as 'self-care' since the rise of the New Right in the 1980s and in direct contravention of the 1978 World Health Organization Alma Ata Declaration that health is a 'fundamental human right and that health policy should acknowledge illness care and the conditions for the creation of health as *collective responsibilities*' (Bella, 2010, p 14, emphasis added). In the UK it was, however, the New Labour government that used the explicit language of patient empowerment, participation, active citizenship in restructuring the welfare state, and one part of this has been through the notion of 'self-care'. Under the rubric of empowerment 'patients were to be "empowered" to engage in self-care and provided with access to the information they needed to ensure health for themselves and their families' (Bella, 2010, p 22). In sharp contrast to earlier feminist notions of empowerment through collective struggle, this translates into health-promotion professionals working with individuals to meet state-sanctioned health-promotion objectives.

The co-option of the language of emancipatory and collective campaigns into the service of the neoliberal agenda of demolishing public health and welfare systems continues. In the policy document that heralded the most draconian dismantling of the NHS since its inception – *Equity and Excellence: Liberating the NHS* (DH, 2010a) by the Coalition government – the term adopted by the international disability movement, 'Nothing about *us* without *us*', was shamelessly appropriated and turned into 'No decision about *me* without *me*' – the slippage from 'us' to 'me' neutralising the collective aspirations of the former and revealing the individualistic intention of the latter.

As the shift to individualised responsibility has intensified, the concept of 'self-care' has become part of the 'solution' to the crisis in NHS funding and the putative unsustainable costs of public health services. This is operationalised through policy discourses and guidance frameworks for professionals that exhort citizens to take more responsibility for their health through the self-management of long-term health conditions and by engaging in 'healthy living' practices. Thus it is not only patients and users of services that need to be persuaded but those who work in the health and social care professions. In the 'position statement' *Self Care – A Real Choice*, issued by the Department of Health and aimed at health and social care professionals and practitioners, we learn that 'Helping people self care represents an exciting opportunity and challenge for the NHS and social care services to empower patients to take more control over their lives' (DH, 2005a, p 1).

Further guidance comes in the accompanying *Self Care Support: A Compendium of Practical Examples Across the Whole System of Health and Social Care* (DH, 2005b), that the role of professionals and practitioners is to support self-care by 'increasing the capacity, confidence and efficacy of the individual for self care and building social capital in the community'. The ways they are expected to carry out this role include providing:

- appropriate and accessible advice. Information and campaigns on lifestyle issues to change behaviours (such as physical activity, healthy eating, other behaviours to sustain well-being and prevent ill-health) and to change the care of minor, acute and long-term conditions
- education of the public and practitioners to change their attitudes and behaviours towards self care. (DH, 2005b, p 5)

The challenge to change health professionals' attitudes has been taken up by the Self Care Forum, a network of self-defined experts from the health professions including doctors, nurses, patient groups, NHS managers, pharmacists, the Department of Health, NHS England and the over-the-counter (OTC) medicines industry. It campaigns to embed self-care within the health service by producing resources and information for health professionals. It understands self-care as a continuum in which at one end 'Healthy Living' represents '100% self-care individual responsibility' and at the opposite end 'In-hospital care' represents '100% medical abdicated responsibility'. It claims that self-care not only empowers the individual but also reduces demand on the NHS and is therefore necessary to 'save' the NHS. On the launch of its mandate *Save our NHS: Time for Action on Self-Care*, it announced: 'The challenge facing the NHS, as a modern means of delivering healthcare, is Darwinian in nature; it must evolve to survive. With an ageing population living longer with long-term conditions, the burden on the NHS will only intensify as greater numbers are affected by ill health' (Self-Care Forum, 2013).

Self-care, then, has become an essential part of neoliberal citizenship responsibility (both for users of services and for those who are professionally employed in them) by using notions of empowerment, choice and control and by drawing on discourses of population ageing and the burden this places on services. The next two sections of the chapter explore how these have been played out in practice with two examples from different areas of policy. First, in relation to the self-management of long-term health conditions and second, in relation to ageing and the promotion of 'active ageing'.

Self-care and 'chronic' health conditions: expert patients

In relation to long-term health conditions (like asthma, diabetes or heart disease), initiatives have been introduced in the UK based on the Chronic Disease Self-Management Programme (CDSMP). Originally developed in Stanford, California, the CDSMP has been adopted in many countries and in England takes the form of the Expert Patients Programme (EPP). It involves training people who have long-term health conditions to develop skills to better self-manage their conditions through a six-week programme led by lay trainers who also have a long-term condition. EPP is underpinned by the assumption that someone with a long-term condition will have developed their own expertise and strategies based on their experience of living with it which will be different to the expertise of the health professionals. Yet this experience is disregarded within the training programme, which is prescriptive and applies 'a model' based on psychological behaviour change, 'reinforcing the medical paradigm' (Wilson et al, 2007, p 427). So it simultaneously acknowledges and denies the expertise of the patient. The 'expert patient' is one who learns 'to behave' in certain ways in relation to their condition and the health professionals they encounter, who takes responsibility to learn to manage the condition so as to become an 'expert': 'Self care involves active citizenry and public engagement; it is also about attitudes and behaviours' (DH, 2005b, p 5).

There are long-standing debates concerning the terms on which patient participation takes place and the extent to which claims that participation leads to empowerment can be justified (Barnes and Cotterell, 2012). The EPP claims to empower the patient to 'feel confident and in control of their life' (NHS Choices web page). Yet participation in EPP is still very much on terms set by medical professionals, and thus the traditional patient–professional relationship is maintained rather than transformed, hidden under the cloak of participation (Wilson et al, 2007).

The basis of EPP is a psychological model of behaviour change that has been widely critiqued because of the importance it attributes to change at the individual level without regard for other structural or cultural variables (Kendall and Rogers, 2007). It sets out normative ways of how individuals should behave, and in the case of EPP patients are expected to conform by following a model prescribed by health professionals. The inference in EPP is that people who have long-term conditions need to modify their behaviour and attitudes in order to better manage their condition. This ignores the ways in which people adapt and learn to live with conditions, and the lived experiences of these processes. As Kendall and Rogers note:

> state sponsored self-management could come to be seen as no more than an attempt to 'hijack' a meaningful concept for the purposes of cost containment, driving down demand for health services through the operationalization of a narrow compliance view of self-management based on a professional educative model. (Kendall and Rogers, 2007, p 140)

Self-care and 'active ageing': ageing as a 'lifestyle' choice

This second example relates to the promotion of healthy lifestyles to prevent costly long-term conditions as people age. As a population group, older people in the UK have been targeted through specific policy objectives linked to the wider 'active ageing' agenda. Arguably, 'active ageing' encompasses a more positive conceptualisation of ageing than a medicalised one, which views ageing as bodily decline and disease, and may well provide a basis to challenge age discrimination and negative stereotyping. However 'active ageing' is a slippery concept, on the one hand used to promote positive images of ageing, on the other hand legitimising neoliberal responses focused on limiting public pensions and healthcare resources.

Within the UK policy 'active ageing' is linked to a public health well-being agenda and to a restructuring of social care provision aimed at reducing costs (DH, 2005c, 2006; HMG, 2010). The policy objectives are expressed through discourses that prioritise the concepts of independence, choice and autonomy and position older people as 'active consumers' of health and care services: 'our overarching objective is to promote well-being and independence. We want to achieve a society where older people are active consumers of public services, exercising control and choice, not passive recipients' (DWP, 2005, p 44).

The National Service Framework for Older People in the UK (DH, 2001a) set 'the promotion of health and active life in older age' as its eighth standard, and subsequent policy emphasised the importance of information and advice on exercise, diet and activity for the achievement of independence and well-being in older age. It has become implicitly linked to notions of self-reliance and avoiding the need for support services and resources, generating a 'sense of obligation' that 'stresses the importance of older people being able to function in ways that best approximate to the ideal of the independent autonomous adult – and for as long as possible' (Lloyd, 2004, p 251).

This policy framework thus conceives the determinants of health as individualistic, and responsibility for 'healthy ageing' is firmly placed with the individual, regardless of all other socioeconomic factors that are known to impact both on health and on the experience of ageing. It fails to acknowledge the now widely accepted view that the life course generally ends in conditions of sickness and dependency, regardless of how successfully an individual has aged healthily (Lloyd, 2012). This increases the binary division between 'independence' and 'dependence', casting those who are in some way dependent on others for their care needs as passive recipients and a 'burden' on the rest of society: 'The responsibility to remain active, which is presented as private self-responsibility towards one's own health, is at the same time the responsibility towards others and the social system, which otherwise faces the burden of a growing number of dependent citizens' (Marhánková, 2011, pp 13–14).

Like other policies and initiatives to promote self-care, 'active ageing' relies on individual consumption choices and behaviours and ignores the wider social and economic contexts that impact on people's capacities to make 'choices' or take individual responsibility. It reframes issues such as social isolation as personal 'risks' that require individual management. Those who experience poverty, social isolation or disability in old age are thus positioned as 'failed citizens' (Laliberte Rudman, 2006) and the state is absolved from responsibility for these as social issues.

Feminist ethics of care: refusing the neoliberal frame

Like all types of care, how self-care is conceptualised is clearly significant to the ways it is practised within health and care interventions. Feminist care ethics has highlighted the importance of paying attention to language in policy discourses as 'modes of governance' in creating hegemonic discourses of care (Sevenhuijsen, 2004) and thus shaping normative understanding of what care is and who has responsibility for it. Neoliberalism is a political rationality that goes beyond its origin in economics. As Doreen Massey notes, it invades our imaginations in its quest to forge a new 'common sense' based on competitive individualism and market relations (Massey, 2013). We can see that the language used in the rationale for self-care – empowerment, choice and control– is a form of linguistic manipulation of arguments made for user involvement by 'self-help' movements. It reflects a move from the collective to the individual, from 'solidarity' of collective self-help towards an extreme 'you are on your own self-care'. The discursive shift from 'voice' to 'choice' is not casual terminology.

In countries that have developed welfare systems, part of the project of neoliberalism must by necessity be about changing the relationship between state and citizen – 'the social contract'. Within current restructuring of health and care systems in developed countries 'self-care' can be understood to be a part of that project, creating a new 'common sense' about what we understand as care, who is responsible for it, what we can do about it, what we expect from the state. It has to tap into ideas about human nature and our beliefs about our 'self' through creating normative ideas that we see in policy discourse – that we are 'independent', we can 'choose' and we 'should' take care of ourselves . For these ideas to become normalised within health and care services, and for it thus to become harder to oppose them or to articulate alternatives, they need to do their 'work' not only on service users but also on workers and professionals who deliver services (see Liveng, Chapter Ten in this volume). Healthcare professionals are now instructed in how to operationalise self-care through personal care planning that 'requires you to adopt a different role to the traditional "diagnoser and treater". The healthcare professional's role is to support individuals to acknowledge, understand and adapt to living with their condition' (Department of Health, 2011, p 3).

Given the context of 'neo-liberal shock doctrine' and the 'assault on every aspect of the welfare state' that has intensified since the 2008 financial crisis (Levitas, 2012, p 326), the arguments emanating from feminist ethics of care are ever more urgent and important. The effects of the shock doctrine are not only discursive shifts in framing 'care' as an individual responsibility but the creation of greater inequalities and social injustice, impacting the most on those already marginalised and vulnerable to market forces and who continue to shoulder most responsibility for care. Feminist ethics of care located in the experiences of care giving and care receiving exposes the gap between the ideology and lived lives.

The reality is that life does involve self-care on a daily basis, and more so in contexts where access to public health and welfare resources is limited or non-existent. But the ways in which this challenge is met are through connectedness with others, in other words, our capacity to be taken care of ourselves is predicated on our connectedness to others. 'Self-care' can only be fully expressed through recognising not only one's own needs for care but also, crucially, that these will be met in relation to others. An ethic of care conceptualises the self that is embedded in relationships with others (from close others, to more distant others such as service providers, paid carers) and therefore autonomy is achievable only in relationship with others.

What the debate about self-care does is take us straight to the question of responsibilities for care and who should have them (see Tronto, Chapter Two in this volume), and the categorical answer from the current proponents of self-care is 'the individual'. The growth and rise of 'self-care' is part and parcel of changing beliefs and cultural attitudes about rights and responsibilities for care in countries that have developed publicly funded welfare systems, so that these come no longer to be regarded as a fundamental part of the social rights of citizenship but as a private, individualised matter. Within an increasingly marketised health and care system this becomes the new 'common sense', not only neutralising beliefs at an individual level but also co-opting some organisations of patients and service users into delivering the 'self-care' agenda. In the case of the UK the decline of social rights to health and welfare is evident in the current break-up of the NHS and the parallel process in relation to 'reforming' the welfare benefit system, which have disproportionately impacted on people with disabilities and people who are carers and women. The transformations are implicated in the distribution of responsibilities for care and are all based on assumptions about individualised responsibility, and framed in moralistic tones of 'scroungers', 'undeserving', 'burden'. The financial crisis and 'austerity' measures provide the perfect 'cover' for implementing a deeply ideological agenda in which the state exonerates itself from its responsibility for providing adequate healthcare for its citizens. It's important to note that in the promotion of self-care it is not just about shifting responsibility *to* the individual, but the shifting *away from* state responsibilities that is at stake.

Self-care is all there is in many places in the world and this looks set to be the pattern in many more places where welfare retrenchment is shifting the boundaries of the social contract. The challenge of self-care is met through people's coming together and this may well provide a form of collective resistance and therefore holds the potential to demand change in the future. But we need to dislodge the idea that self-care is about individual empowerment and choice and to use care ethics as a critical tool to refuse the neoliberal frame and the unequal distribution of responsibilities for care that it produces.

FIVE

Care ethics, intersectionality and poststructuralism

Nicki Ward

Introduction

Notions of identity, intersectionality and poststructuralism all involve a consideration of what it is to be 'other'. As Simone de Beauvoir suggests:

> 'Otherness is a fundamental category of human thought. Thus it is that no group even sets itself up as the One without at once setting up the Other' (1972, p 17).

While notions of 'the one' and 'the other' still inform understandings of identity, the categories that constitute oneness or otherness have become increasingly complex. The rise of poststructural ways of understanding the world and the development of our understanding of intersectionality have, since their emergence in the latter part of the 20th century, become increasingly significant. The disruption of the old sureties of identity through the interrogation of binary distinctions, along with the shrinking world of cross-cultural relations, migration and globalisation, have all served to demonstrate the myth of the presumption that identity was fixed and representative of a particular and immutable relationship to social structures.

Here, the concept of poststructuralism accorded with the critiques developed by black feminist thinkers in relation to intersectionality, which illustrated that the experience of women was not a homogenous one, but was differentiated across lines of 'race', class and power. So, as Crenshaw (1991, p 1242) notes, the concern was not that identity politics failed to address and rise above issues of difference, but that it was inclined to ignore or conflate the differences between groups. The argument for an intersectional analysis was that the experiences of black women could be fully understood only by considering how experiences of race and gender intersected in those women's lives, rather than by treating them as separate categories. The poststructuralist critique of essentialism and homogenising notions of identity was seen to offer a challenge to universalism and to 'open up new possibilities for the construction of self and the assertion of agency' (hooks, 1991, p 28).

The ability to think intersectionally requires openness, awareness of fluidity and the willingness to interrogate power (Crenshaw, cited in Adewunmi, 2014). It is this openness and fluidity that has led to the consideration of different lines of intersectional analysis. While intersectionality is no longer limited to considerations of race, class and gender, and may now be expanded to consider other dimensions of difference, such as sexuality, disability and age, the critical analysis offered by theories of intersectionality is, nevertheless, still 'at the heart of feminist theory and practice' (Yuval Davis, 2006a, p 194) and, as such, it is important to consider how it relates to a feminist ethic of care.

Hankivsky (2014) has suggested both that care ethics may have something to lend to the theory of intersectionality and that intersectionality also lends itself to a development of care ethics. This chapter develops that notion by considering how the two theories might complement each other; not only in exploring the different theoretical and philosophical positions, but also in how they might expand our understanding of the lived realities of care, identity and diversity.

Identity and care ethics: a symbiotic relationship?

Identity is about belonging, it is forged through processes in which we develop an understanding of ourselves in relation to other people, our commonalities and the attributes we share, but it is also that which marks us out as different. However, identity is also something that shifts and changes as we move through life. It is impacted on by wider discourses that not only give name to different identities and set boundaries around who can claim them, but also influences which of these are seen as positive or negative within different spatial and temporal locations.

As such, identity is formed and experienced through relationships of power and knowledge. Identity may be seen as something that is subjectively located, understood as personal expression of identity, or as socially ascribed. Seen subjectively, it is something that sits within us, as represented in the phrase 'sense of self', while ascribed identity derives from the labelling, beliefs and assumptions that attach to different discourses of identity. While this may be a useful analytical distinction that enables a consideration of the different components of identity and its formation, it is also important to note that the relationship between these different aspects of identity is also a part of the process of identity formation; a relationship that is both complex and subtle (Layder, 2004; Wetherell, 2008). Subjective understandings of our selves do not develop in isolation, they develop in relation to the characteristics, attributes and stereotypes ascribed to different identity positions. We are, as Tronto notes, constantly working through, in and away 'from relationships with others' (2013, p 31). It is through our relationship with others, and also the interaction – or relationship – between self and ascribed identity, that we come to understand ourselves, our differences and similarities, and our positioning. Subjectivity and social ascription are not divisible from each other, they are part of the practice of identity that is 'absolutely integral to the very construction and definition of social categories and their cultural imagining' (Wetherell, 2008, p 77).

There are many parallels between an understanding of identity as relationally constructed and the ontological perspective of a critical ethic of care. A critical ethics of care adopts a relational ontology. From this position our lives and our understanding of the world are understood as formed through relationships; relationships that are not always or only positive but that may also construct and enact power and knowledge in ways that can be damaging and exclusionary (Robinson, 1999). People and the problems that they are perceived to present derive from processes of power. The relational ontology encapsulated by care ethics can alert us not only to the subjective particularities of the experience as lived, but also to the creation and reification of those social power relations. In this sense care ethics can be seen as a 'phenomenology of moral life that recognises that addressing moral problems involves first, an understanding of identities, relationships, and contexts' (Robinson, 1999, p 31).

Care ethics then, is an important framework, through which to understand and explore complex identity positions. At the same time, identity is an important concept for a critical ethics of care. The way that people's identities are constructed and positioned can mean that their needs for care and their roles within relationships of care are either given credence, marginalised or, in some cases, rendered invisible. What I am suggesting in this chapter is that we can perceive of the relationship between a critical ethic of care and poststructuralist understandings of identity as symbiotic.

In the sections that follow I consider in more depth the complementary connections between care ethics, identity and intersectionality to consider two issues: firstly, how care ethics might help to locate and engage with subjective experiences of intersectionality and difference, and secondly, how intersectionality might help up to understand the emergence of new identities of care.

Poststructuralism, intersectionality and a critical ethics of care

Poststructuralist theory challenges grand narratives that function to normalise or homogenise experience and obscure the historical, cultural, geographic and social differences that serve to construct people's experience in different ways. A poststructural way of thinking is one that interrogates and undermines binary oppositions, challenging approaches to identity that present it as homogenised and grounded in naturalised, biological differences. Because poststructuralism challenges notions of fixedness, including 'unified subjectivity and centred theories of power' (Weedon, 1999, p 100), it has lent itself to the critiques of identity politics made by queer theorists and black feminists (among others), opening up new ways to consider experiences of identity and how these intersect.

Intersectionality is at the heart of difference. It is something that marks out both the sense of self that is shared with others and its points of divergence, through the characteristics of gender, ethnicity, race, sexuality, (dis)ability, religion, culture, age and so on. However, it is not simply an additive formula for understanding identity, but one that seeks to explain and understand the combined effect of cross-cutting intersectional experience and how the subject positions involved may serve to constitute each other. Identities become reconfigured through these myriad lenses, across different cultural, temporal and geographic spaces. As Williams (2002) argues, for example, 'the hybridity of cultures hangs on the hyphens which join Black to British, Scottish to Asian or African to Caribbean' (p 515). Experiences of identity are not simply reflections of different social positions, but derive from being differently positioned 'along an axis of power' (Yuval Davis, 2006b, p 199). In this context intersectionality is an 'analytical tool' that can challenge the traditional reified approaches to identity politics and understandings of social stratification (Yuval Davis, 2006a, p 201).

Yuval Davis (2011) has argued that citizenship is always constructed in relation to intersecting social divisions that arise through a process of othering and differentiation. Such processes can obscure our view of the person, and can also shift and change in different contexts as power plays out differently. The 'concrete *experiences of* oppression ... [are] ... always constructed and intermeshed with other social divisions'

(Yuval Davis, 2006a, p 195; my emphasis). To understand poststructural, intersectional identities is not, and should not be, a solely philosophical exercise. Discursive constructions have a real impact on people's lives (Ward, 2009). When we fail to understand and engage with people in all of their complexity, we compromise their ability to be a whole person in all of the activities of their life. As one woman notes when discussing her own intersectional identity as a lesbian feminist who also experiences mental health difficulties:

> 'It's like other people are always trying to make you separate stuff out, not for you but for them … You know are you doing this as a woman or as a lesbian or as somebody with a mental health problem or what and it's like but they are all me, they are all part of me. You know that's bloody where lies madness if you ask me … People will try and go oh that's not relevant and that's not relevant but you can't sort people out into bits.' (Amy, cited in Ward, 2005)

Intersectional identities do not respond well to normative judgements about rights because such normative judgements tend to focus on one dimension of identity at a time and rely on generalisations about how people are affected by something or what is needed. Moral philosophy has historically focused on the notion of what is the right action to take, and on creating a set of principles that will enable people to make the right moral choices. However, in a world marked out by difference and diversity what is right, and for whom, is likely to be different in the very different subjective contexts in which we live. It is in this context that care ethicists argue that a more contextual and situated ethical engagement is needed (Sevenhuijsen, 1998; Robinson, 1999;). The problem of a notion of justice, or of codified rights, as impartial, even if it is possible to have an objective set of rules and principles that define justice and rights, is that they become partial when applied to different people's lives (Hankivsky, 2004). In this way a policy or rule that is seen as generic, and that may be premised on 'good care' for one particular group, can actually serve to exclude, particularly in the context of intersectional identities. So, for example, campaigns and services for what are perceived as gender-specific cancers such as prostate or cervical cancer may exclude and deter trans people from seeking support (Fish, 2006).

This should not, however, be seen as an argument for individual particularity. Rather, it is an acknowledgement of the danger of decontextualising people's lives and the importance of analysing the way that different processes may produce different and discriminatory experiences. Critiques of a feminist ethic of care, as they originated with the work of Carol Gilligan, have suggested that it is partial, and does not acknowledge aspects of intersectionality with class, race and so on (Hankivsky, 2014; see Robinson, 1999 for further discussion). However, it is also important to see it as a product of its time; an incomplete theory, as most are, but not one without merit. The point is not to reject it, but to take the principles and to apply them in a way that does acknowledge the historical and social specificity of the original. Gilligan (1982) herself suggested that a care ethic needed a contextual sensitivity. In considering intersectional identities such a contextual sensitivity can enable us to identify the ways that temporal, spatial and political locations, along with different social and cultural understandings, may all serve to construct different intersectional experiences of identity that in turn influence peoples' lived realities.

Many of the critiques that argue that care ethics carry with them a danger of essentialising women and reinforcing the gender stereotypes that constrain women to the private sphere are, I would argue, taking the principles as 'feminine', rather than seeing them as feminist principles that seek to challenge the hegemonic masculinity of traditional frames of reference. As Tronto (1993) argues, a feminist approach broadens our understanding of what it means to care, bringing it out of the private realm and centralising it within the lives of everyone. It is in centralising care within people's lived realities that I believe care ethics has a particular strength for exploring and understanding intersectionality. Further critiques have suggested that care ethics are not conceptually inclusive and do not attend adequately to questions of power (Hankivsky, 2014). However, a political ethic of care as developed by Tronto (1993, 2013) does, I would suggest, do this, by explicitly attending to the role of political structures in framing and valuing (or devaluing) care and emphasising the importance of these issues to all of our lives. Our personal lives are affected by the political, and the impact of the political, as encapsulated in public and social policy, has differential impact related to aspects of identity and intersectionality. Care ethics, then, are not in themselves universalising as some critics might suggest, except perhaps in the understanding of the universality of interdependence and the importance of interrelationality in everyone's lives.

While it may be the case that care ethics has rarely engaged with intersectionality on a theoretical level, drawing on a political ethic of care does offer a way to address some of the challenges of intersectionality, particularly in terms of 'identifying and articulating the synergistic effects of interlocking structures of power' (Hankivsky, 2014, p 260). Care ethics explicitly attends to the context of the situation and the impact of power relationships in order to understand the experience of the people involved so as to help inform responses that are located in people's lived realities. As such, it has the ability to recognise the axes of power that are ever present that may impact differently on people, depending on the fluidity of identities and subject positions. This is demonstrated through the many experiences that care ethics has been used to consider and illuminate as, for example, in discussions of gender location and class (Peters et al, 2010), gender and age, (Lloyd, 2010), gender, work and care (McDowell, 2004) and transgender practices of care (Hines, 2007). In the context of understanding intersectional experience it is this recognition of the social axes of power that is of political importance (Yuval Davis, 2006a).

A critical ethic of care acknowledges that ethical decisions need to be situated in order to enable us to know and to judge in context, as Sevehuijsen argues: 'only attention to specificity and contextuality can keep us from expecting ethics to be a source of absolute normative truth' (1998, p 16). When applied to intersectionality this specificity and contextuality can enable an analysis that identifies the synergistic effects of power and the way that these impact on lived lives, by working from, and being attentive to, the subjective experiences of those affected by such structures.

Carer and cared for: new intersections of identity

Identity, as a basis of our understanding of ourselves and others and of our relational positioning, is not monolithic. As Stuart Hall argued: 'Identities are ... increasingly fragmented and fractured; never singular but multiply constructed across different, often intersecting and antagonistic discourses, practices and positions' (Hall, 1996, p 4). Not only are identities not monolithic but, as poststructuralism demonstrates, the multiple constructions of identity mean that new and emerging subject positions are always becoming articulated and acknowledged. The challenges made to identity politics by those who feel excluded and marginalised within such conceptions have led to the constant rearticulation of new and shifting forms of identity. My own engagement with queer communities over the past three decades – and the way that these groups have been named – provides a useful example. During the 1980s many support groups and community organisations were labelled as being LG – for lesbians and gay men. The early 1990s started to see debates among these groups for the addition of the B, to indicate the inclusivity of those who defined as bisexual. Subsequent debates followed for the inclusion of the T, to represent inclusivity of the trans community and, in some circles, the specific inclusion of the I to distinguish people who were intersex. The arrival of Queer theory led to further developments, with some adding a Q as in LGBTQI, and others using the Q as a representation of gender and sexual diversity. This not only demonstrates the shifting and sometimes transient aspects of identity – queer, for example, has been and is experienced as both stigmatising and liberating – but is also representative of a somewhat additive approach to identity.

Care ethicists have argued that care is something that concerns us all and that will touch all of our lives (Tronto, 1993). While this may be a truism, the ways in which we are involved in care are neither homogenous nor equal (Williams, 2002, p 510). This is why it is helpful to consider care, and the identities and subject positions associated with it, through the lenses of poststructuralism and intersectionality. The relationship between care and gender is well rehearsed and this has been further explicated in relation to gender and class (Tronto, 2013), gender and ethnicity (Williams, 2002) and age (Lloyd, 2010; Holland, 2010) and has begun to be considered by others in relation to disability (Ward, 2011; Fudge Schormans, Chapter Fourteen in this volume) and sexuality (Price, 2010; Willis et al, 2011). What has been less apparent, however, is how we might understand care and the different subject positions of carer and cared for as emerging constructions of identity that themselves are experienced intersectionally. From an intersectional perspective it is important that we think broadly about identity and 'remain open to new and emerging aspects of identity and intersectional experience (Hankivsky, 2014, p 258, citing Thorvaldsdottir, 2007). Here I aim to consider how 'carer' and 'cared for' are representative of emergent identities that need to be explored and understood through an intersectional lens.

Barnes notes that the identity of 'carers' as a social group was established by the 'emergence of the carers movement' (Barnes, 2006, p 136). The way that such social groups or categories emerge and the way in which they become embedded within policy and practice may differ. For some it has been based on the campaigns of new social movements, while for others their creation has been stimulated by the establishment of particular categories within policy and practice, and the need to claim these subject positions in order to access services. But each of these emergent identities 'enter into the social field as primary units of social representation and organisation … located in the operations of power' (Anthias, 2013, p 8). This can be seen in the way in which categories of 'carer' and 'service user' have emerged and become embedded in policy and practice within the UK, particularly in the fields of social work, social care and health. Social policy in this area has, increasingly, included a requirement to involve service users and carers in the development and delivery of services and professional education (Levin, 2004; Needham and Carr, 2009). I am certainly not seeking to argue here that this is not appropriate; I would agree that those who use services and are affected most by them should be involved in their development and delivery. However, it is also important to consider the ways that such inclusion can reify certain subject positions while at the same time contributing to 'intersectional invisibility' (Crenshawe, 2000 cited in Anthias, 2013). Thus, for example, it may be difficult for those who have already been defined within policy as being vulnerable and in need of care, such as people with learning disabilities, or children who are in the care of public services, to also be seen as carers (Holland, 2010; Ward, 2011). Within this situated context their roles as carers, constituted through their identities as vulnerable, result in a process that can render this aspect of their identity invisible and can obscure any related needs. (see Ward, N., Chapter Thirteen in this volume).

Not only does the way in which one defines oneself, or is defined by others, have an impact on belonging, it can also have an impact on life chances and determine the grounds on which one can participate socially, culturally and politically (Anthias, 2013). The active dimension of identity is apparent not only in the ways that individuals and groups express themselves, but also in broader political contexts. In turn these affect the way that people are able to present themselves and the identity positions they can claim (Sevenhuijsen, 1998, p 30). Legal and policy texts can be seen as discursive spaces within which subject positions are created and through which people may be included or excluded in particular ways. As such, they either enable or constrain human agency (Sevenhuijsen, 1998, p 31). Yuval Davis echoes this and notes that hegemonic discourses not only 'render invisible experiences of more marginal members', but also construct beliefs about the 'right way' to be a part of the group (2006a, p 195). From my own experience of working as a paid support worker and of managing residential support services I know that in the UK it is widely accepted that personal and intimate care should be delivered by someone of the same gender, except perhaps where there is already an established relationship of intimacy such as that between spouses, and this is acknowledged in policy and practice guidance (Carnaby and Cambridge, 2006; Surrey and Borders NHS Partnership, 2007). However, for men who identify as gay, and who are identified as such by professionals, the rules and norms pertaining to gender assumptions can be applied differently, as for example in a situation where professionals explicitly articulate that it's OK for a 'gay' grandson who lives with his frail grandmother to see her naked and tend to her intimate care needs because he is gay (Willis et al, 2011).

The provision and receipt of care is often conceived of as a resource, the access to which, like other resources, is determined by social relations and by socioeconomic and political power (Sevenhuijsen, 1998, p 23). The emergence of the identity of carer illustrates this, drawing on economic constructions of the value of care to society and engaging a political voice – but only for some. Carer has become a category, and claiming this particular subject position or identity can be important in gaining access to services and support (Barnes, 2011b). However, as Yuval Davis (2006a) observes, such categorical attributes can be used to construct boundaries of self and other and determine who has entitlement to resources.

Care ethics not only helps to understand, unpack and identify the subjectively lived experience but also, through the political lens, to understand how identities and subject positions become constructed, reified and acknowledged – or rendered invisible – within policy. Social divisions are formulated in experiential, intersubjective, organisational and representational terms (Yuval Davis, 2006a) that can be expressed through politics and policy. Social policy creates certain subject positions in order to organise and deliver public services, and those who wish to access these services will have to claim – and prove – their 'entitlement' to occupy these positions. People with learning disabilities may be required to take an IQ test in order to prove their entitlement to specialist educational provision, or people who are seeking asylum will have to prove they have a well-founded fear of persecution or have been subjected to human rights abuses. Such ascribed and imposed identities can in turn add to intersectional experience. So women with learning disabilities regularly have their parenting capacity questioned and find themselves subject to child protection procedures (Booth and Booth, 2005). Because care ethics focuses on care giver and care receiver and on their relationship it opens up our ability to be alert to the way that these subject positions create new and different intersectional experiences of identity and care.

So, both carers and those perceived as the 'cared for' need to position themselves in particular ways in order to access support. However, the discourses that contribute to the understanding of these different subject positions can create boundaries between group belonging, in such a way that it can be difficult to claim multiple intersecting identities. A recent consultation by the Health and Care Professions Council in the UK (the regulatory body for health and care professionals) sought feedback on developing a standard to guide service user involvement and, as part of this, consulted on the definition. A significant number of the responses argued that carers should be categorised and acknowledged separately from service users. Arguments included the idea that carers should be separately but equally valued, that they had interlinked but different perspectives and that they were recognised separately in legislation, policy and common terminology (HCPC, 2013, p 19). What such debates do is construct and reinforce the binary distinction between 'carer' and 'cared for'.

Thinking about care, about who cares and how, is a moral, social and political issue that requires exploration of the way that different roles and relationships are constructed within the broader sociopolitical contexts (Tronto, 1993; Robinson, 1999, p 33). From an intersectional perspective it is important to consider not only the construction of personal positions, identities and political value, but also the specific socioeconomic political experience of those involved in caring relationships at that point in time (Yuval Davis, 2006a). From a care ethics perspective we need to be attentive to the way that different moral, social and political contexts, located within particular hegemonic cultural representations, not only are experienced intersectionally but also can serve to construct the ways in which certain intersectional identities can be seen and others cannot. The identity of carer may be seen to more 'naturally' or visibly intersect with some identities than others, and in the context of the identities of 'carer' and 'cared for' the two are often seen as immutable.

Conclusion

This chapter has considered the way that an ethic of care may lend itself to furthering an understanding of lived experiences of intersectionality, while also arguing that intersectionality can deepen our awareness of experiences of care. 'Intersectionality' does not refer to a particular state of being or location, but rather to a process that needs to be understood as a relational dynamic (Anthias, 2013). It involves the relationship between people, assessments of sameness and difference and diversity, but also the relationship between individuals and the sociopolitical structures experienced relationally. A critical ethic of care that emphasises the importance of attending with care to a person's subjective experience, of understanding this as something created in relationship and of locating this within the wider context of social power relations has much to offer to our understanding of experiences of intersectionality.

At the same time, as Tronto has argued, 'any account of care that is not pluralistic will end up imposing bad care on some, and thus impinging on some people's liberties' (Tronto, 2013, p xiv). While care may be all pervasive in the sense that it affects all of our lives, it does not affect them all equally or consistently. And if we adopt approaches to care, and the subject positions within relationships of care, that are constructed along the lines of binary distinctions or universalising principles, then we are in danger of imposing bad care on some. At some point in our lives we will all be carers and we will all be cared for; we may fulfil these roles successively or even simultaneously, and as such we need to be aware of our interdependencies and the networks and webs of care that we inhabit (Barnes, Chapter Three; Williams, 2004a). Considered intersectionally, these positions can be seen as being constituted through other aspects of identity and also as constituting each other, in a way that is linked to the hierarchies of power (Anthias, 2013). Caring is marked by social and cultural values and formations; if we are to ensure that we do not 'distort social reality' (Anthias, 2013, p 68), then we need to recognise the experience of intersectionality within this.

SIX

Care ethics and indigenous values: political, tribal and personal

Amohia Boulton and Tula Brannelly

Introduction

In this chapter we ask if it is possible that care ethics be informed and supported by values and practices that are common or foundational to indigenous knowledges. Indigenous cultures, despite their heterogeneity and diversity, construct societies and conduct relationships in accordance to values and practices that are often the antithesis of neoliberalism, as does care ethics. We have written elsewhere about the centrality of humanness and relationality within te ao Māori (Māori world-view) (Brannelly, Boulton and Te Hiini, 2013). In this chapter we extend this discussion by considering broader political questions that echo and relate between care ethics and other world-views. Amohia is a Māori woman with tribal affiliations to Ngāti Ranginui, Ngai te Rangi and Ngāti Pukenga in the Bay of Plenty and Ngāti Mutunga in Taranaki, and Tula is a Pākehā woman, a citizen of Aotearoa/New Zealand, having migrated from the UK. We base our observations on three elements of Māori values and practice: whanaungatanga (kinship), kaitiakitanga (guardianship) and manaakitanga (care). Relational, collective values and practices are relevant to other indigenous cultures and, where possible, we draw on Aboriginal (Australia), and Canadian First Nations knowledge. Key issues resulting from colonisation that are hotly contested in colonised societies are health inequalities, land rights and environmentalism, and thus we use these to illustrate the on-going challenge to neoliberal health and social policies and the resonance with care ethics.

The broad political questions posed by care ethics that are of particular relevance to colonised societies relate to care and justice in terms of the responses to indigenous peoples as marginalised communities within settler colonies. This positioning raises questions regarding privileged (ir)responsibility for attentiveness to indigenous peoples. In indigenous cultures and in care ethics, the moral boundaries of care and politics are intertwined rather than divorced into separate spheres. Past injustices and the hurt and harms that result from them are acknowledged in the present context of health and social care provision, and other pressing issues for indigenous people, such as land rights. The embedded market philosophy in health and social care provision that fails to appreciate, capture or adequately fund the caring activities within iwi (tribes) is also questioned. The knowledges and practices of indigenous cultures relevant to care ethics are a long tradition of 'species activities of maintaining and sustaining the world' that include relationships with the past and responsibilities to the future; and collective interdependence as an expectation of societal responsibility that structures and governs relationships and responsibilities.

We do not claim expertise in all indigenous knowledge, nor seek to justify those knowledges using Western colonial concepts. We are interested in initiating a conversation about the power and strength of indigenous knowledges, as an acknowledgement of the previous harms that have been caused to indigenous peoples through processes of colonisation where languages have become extinct, populations have been decimated and on-going struggles to connect people and land remain current. In our discussion of indigeneity, we acknowledge that our generalisations do not adequately capture diversity, but are necessary for the brevity of discussion. The United Nations (2010, p 3) identified that no universally accepted international definition of indigenous people exists, and provided the following explanation:

> indigenous people are descendants of peoples who inhabited the land prior to colonisation, and who possess distinct social, economic and political systems, languages, cultures and beliefs and are determined to maintain and develop this distinct identity; they exhibit strong attachments to their ancestral lands and the natural resources contained therein; and/or they belong to non-dominant groups of a society and identify themselves as indigenous people.

Australia, Canada and Aotearoa/New Zealand were settled at different times, and with different consequences, one of which is that Aotearoa has a Treaty (of Waitangi) that ensures a direct relationship between the indigenous population and the British Crown. The Treaty of Waitangi has widely accepted principles: partnership, protection and self-determination, that influence and inform the relationship between the Crown (government) and Māori, and that are challenged, for example, through land-rights hearings in the Treaty of Waitangi tribunal. This was not the case in Australia (where earlier colonisers professed *terra nullius*) or in Canada (where colonisers settled even earlier), both of whose Aboriginal and First Nations peoples are in the process of establishing treaties (Gott, 2011). The timing and initial interactions between the colonisers and colonised were important in setting the future of relations in those countries and have a direct relationship to the kinds of outcomes apparent today.

Core Māori values that can inform an ethic of care

Māori, as the indigenous people of Aotearoa, share a similar colonial history to many other Aboriginal or indigenous peoples the world over. Arguably, it was as a consequence of the process of colonisation that the collective term 'Māori' was applied to the indigenous peoples of Aotearoa (Royal, 2011). Prior to colonisation, Māori were a tribal people, identifying ourselves through whakapapa (genealogy) to one (usually male) eponymous ancestor, or to a physical location. Hence the tribe named Ngāti Mutunga are the descendants of ancestor Mutunga and others who lived in a particular part of Aotearoa. In addition to descent lines that originate from those who took part in the great voyaging migrations thought to have occurred some 800 years ago, tribes may also have origin stories in which ancestors came from the natural environment, directly from the land or the waters.

Prior to contact with Europeans, Māori society was held together by a series of rules, conventions and customs collectively known as tikanga, which operated to keep members safe, healthy and thriving. Hirini Moko Mead (2003, p 12) defines tikanga as the set of beliefs associated with practices and procedures to be followed in conducting the affairs of a group or individual. Derived from the accumulated knowledge of generations of Māori, tikanga determined how people would interact not only with members of their tribe but also with visitors, strangers and with the wider world. Tikanga also directed how individuals and the collective were to conduct themselves during different ceremonies or rites of passage such as during pregnancy, childbirth or when a person passed away, and structured the ritual of encounter.

The connections to both the physical world and the spiritual world were deep and abiding. Māori understood the physical world (land, rivers, lakes, seas) as extensions of their whakapapa or genealogical roots. The land was the physical manifestation of Papatuānuku, the Earth Mother, and the sky was the father of all creation, Ranginui. Rangi and Papa gave birth to all living creatures that inhabited the physical realm. Māori and the creatures we shared our world with were related through whakapapa or genealogical links to Ranginui and Papatuānuku.

For Māori, the spirit world was (and is) simply another plane of existence, albeit one that demands considerable respect. This world was inhabited by, among others, those ancestors who had passed on before. Thus, for Māori, ancestors were never truly 'gone'; rather, they inhabited a realm that was different to that inhabited by the living. The closeness between the two realms meant that for Māori, ancestors and ancestral wisdom were always close at hand, and time or the temporal dimension was not neatly segregated into notions of past, present and future. Māori acceptance of the 'nearness' of our ancestors persists today and can be seen, for example, in our attitudes to matakite, those who possess second sight, who experience hearing of voices or have visitations from ancestors. Far from being an aberration, matakite are regarded as gifted and able to communicate with beings and entities from these other planes, including those who have passed on. One impact of colonisation is the introduction and dominance of Western medical systems, including psychiatry, which view this phenomenon as psychosis, and this has, for some, had the consequence of incorrect diagnosis and harms related to institutionalisation and forced treatment (Bidois, 2011).

Concepts of connectedness and interdependence remain crucial to how Māori view the world, make sense of physical phenomena and adapt and survive as a people. This sense of interdependence, the adherence to the strength of the collective, an ancient relationship with a defined territory, and the understanding that humans are inextricably linked to the natural world are beliefs held in common by many indigenous peoples (Helin, 2006; Boulton, 2007).

Despite the ravages Māori people faced through colonisation, contemporary Māori have managed, for the most part, to retain tribal identity, if not the lands and territories to which we were and are so inextricably linked. While there are a large number of so-called 'urban' Māori who, as a consequence of colonisation and subsequent policies of assimilation, have lost both contact with their tribal lands and knowledge of their whakapapa, the majority of Māori today know their tribal links. Furthermore, in a process of decolonisation and cultural revitalisation, many are taking active steps to reclaim traditional Māori knowledges, customs and practices in fields as diverse as the arts, oratory, ceremony and health and healing.

The results of this cultural revitalisation have been many and varied, having been facilitated to some degree by the Crown's acknowledgement of its responsibilities under the Treaty of Waitangi and thus supported by government funding. For instance, in the field of education, institutions to teach te reo Māori (the Māori language), drawing on Māori epistemology and pedagogy, now exist for learners of all ages, from pre-school children through to adult learners in tertiary settings. Māori cultural revitalisation has also made its mark in the health, well-being and caring sectors, with the development and promulgation through health and social services of Māori models of health and well-being (for example, Te Whare Tapa Wha); in the environment sector, through the adoption of Māori concepts into resource management strategies and environmental policy; in broadcasting, where Māori have secured the rights to part of the broadcasting 'spectrum'; and at the interface of economic development and law with the development of mechanisms to 'manage' the land titles and other assets (for example fisheries) held in collective ownership.

Irrespective of the field of endeavour or sector of concern, what Māori as indigenous people are able to bring to the table is a set of values that have endured in the face of colonisation, population decimation[1] and major societal change. These are values which provide an alternative to the neoliberal push to extend the market mechanism into every facet of community (Bargh, 2007); values which form the very foundation of our society. These values include whanaungatanga, manaakitanga and kaitiakitanga, each of which is explained below.

Whanaungatanga

Whanaungatanga is defined as 'a relationship through shared experiences and working together which provides people with a sense of belonging. It develops as a result of kinship rights and obligations, which also serve to strengthen each member of the kin group. It also extends to others to whom one develops a close familial, friendship or reciprocal relationship' (see maoridictionary.co.nz). O'Carroll (2013) explains whanaungatanga, or the process of attaining and maintaining relationships, is one by which people collectively socialise and engage in enhancing their relationships. McNatty and Roa observe the central place of whanaungatanga in the Māori world-view, evidenced by the fact that it is referred to, directly or indirectly, in a great diversity of contexts, where its exact meaning emerges through association rather than explicit definition (McNatty and Roa, 2002, p 90). Ritchie (1992) describes whanaungatanga as the 'basic cement that holds things Māori together' (p 67). Whanaungatanga is central to a Māori world-view, as it draws a range of duties, rights, responsibilities, obligations and values together in one concept. More than simply a linear relationship between one person and another, whanaungatanga acknowledges and takes account of the past, recognises the present and seeks a foundation for the future. In the extended family setting, the purpose of whanaungatanga is to cement relationships and duties and ensure that the bonds of kinship are constantly reviewed, renewed and strengthened.

Whanaungatanga involves protocols, histories, genealogy (whakapapa) and role responsibilities and duties. In writing about one person's experience of whanaungatanga, McNatty and Roa observe that whanaungatanga requires us to immediately understand, and respond to, a complex set of interrelationships – social, cultural, spiritual and ancestral – 'a web of inter-related aspects of life processes' (McNatty and Roa, 2002, p 91). More than simply extending the hand of friendship and making 'connections' or 'networking', whanaungatanga establishes the protocols or ground rules by which interaction can occur.

Whakawhanaungatanga, the process of establishing these relationships, has been described as a traditional and a contemporary strength for Māori (Lemon, no date). Through whakawhanaungatanga, Māori are able to make links and connections beyond their extended family to other people, primarily through whakapapa (genealogical connections), but also through shared histories and experiences. The importance of whanaungatanga is understood best when considered in the light of how Māori were able to survive as a people in an unforgiving natural environment, and when beset by colonisation, war and disease. The concept of whanaungatanga is closely linked to that of whakapapa, in that people are more likely to be able to build and sustain relationships if they have an understanding of their own genealogical connections and can use this knowledge to demonstrate the connections and linkages with another person's origins of tribe, sub-tribe, people and lands.

Manaakitanga

The concepts of manaaki – to support or take care of, to give hospitality to, to protect and look out for – and manaakitanga – the act of providing support, hospitality, protection and care – are fundamental to Māori culture, providing clear guidelines for how people, but particularly visitors, should be treated. Roa and Tuaupiki observe that manaakitanga forms the basis of all well-intentioned human interaction and refers to the obligation to respect the 'other', whether the other be living, dead or passed on, or even non-human. The act of manaakitanga also refers to nurturing and fostering relationships and treating the other with care and respect (Roa and Tuaupiki, 2005).

To understand the true nature of the concept, and indeed the obligation that providing manaaki demands of those who offer it and those who receive it, it is necessary to understand that the word manaaki is comprised of two separate words: 'mana', referring to a person's status, 'power', authority or influence; and 'aki', meaning to encourage or support, or to challenge where necessary. Manaakitanga, the act of providing manaaki to someone, therefore encompasses values such as generosity and kindness, hospitality and a responsibility to look after and care for people. A key component of manaakitanga is the idea of elevating your own and others' mana (authority and status) through sharing of material and non-material goods (Gifford and Boulton, forthcoming). As Spiller notes, reciprocity lies at the heart of manaakitanga and it is through service that we are able to enhance the mana of others (Spiller et al, 2011).

Professor Manuka Henare (geoteachers.blogspot.co.nz) observes that

> manaakitanga relates to the finer qualities of people, rather than just to their material possessions. It is the principle of the quality of caring, kindness, hospitality and showing respect for others. To exhibit manaakitanga is to raise ones [sic] mana (manaaki) through generosity.

Manaakitanga, by definition, then, encompasses notions of aroha (love) and mutual respect and, when offered appropriately, enhances the status of both the giver and the receiver. Manaakitanga transforms mana through acts of generosity that enhance all, that produce well-being and create 'a climate whereby the mana of all players is elevated' (Durie, 2001, p 83). Uplifting the mana of others in turn nourishes one's own mana.

Kaitiakitanga

The terms kaitiakitanga (guardianship) and kaitiaki (to guard or protect when used as a verb, or a guardian or steward when used as a noun) are most commonly used when discussing environmental protection, natural resource management and conservation, as, traditionally, the role of the Kaitiaki was to protect certain places and/or natural resources. One of the first scholars to write about this traditional institution described the Kaitiaki as a tribal custodian or guardian. The writer observed, however, that to understand the role of the Kaitiaki one has to understand the intricacies of Māori society. Accordingly, the concept of kaitiaki does not stand alone but, rather:

> it is part of a complex social, cultural, economic and spiritual system that has been established though long tribal associations with land and waters. To know Kaitiaki is to know the Māori world – the tribal structures of iwi (tribes), hapū (sub-tribes), whanau (extended family), tangata whenua (people of the land), manawhenua (authority and title over land and other resources), ahi kaa (people born in their tribal area who have always resided on their traditional lands), Kaitiaki, kaumatua (older men), kuia (older women), tohunga (knowledge-holders), whanaunga (relatives) – and that these make up a pulsating thriving Māori community. (Minhinnick, 1989, p 1)

Later writers have expanded on the concept of kaitiaki, illuminating the practices associated with kaitiakitanga, or guardianship. According to Whangapirita, Awatere and Nikora (2003) the term kaitiaki refers to:

> the responsibility that certain entities, not exclusively people, have to protect and guard the mauri (life principle) of particular groups, objects, resources, traditions, practices and places ... The Kaitiaki role is not a process of ownership but an individual and collective role to safeguard ngā taonga tuku iho (the treasures handed down) for the present and future generations. (Whangapirita et al, 2003, p 6)

Kawharu (2000) notes that what kaitiakitanga entails in practice may differ between tribes or even among members of the same tribe. However, despite differences in how kaitaikitanga is applied, there are a set of essential features which characterise the concept, namely that kaitiatakitanga integrates beliefs pertaining to spiritual, human and environmental spheres. Values such as tapu and noa (the sacred and profane); mauri (the life force); rangatiratanga (the right to exercise authority or self-determination); manawhenua (customary authority over land); and rahui (a temporary ritual prohibition on an area, resource or stretch of water) are all bound up in the concept of kaitiakitanga (Marsden and Henare, 1992).

Kaitiakitanga also embraces social protocols associated with hospitality, reciprocity and obligation (manaaki, tuku and utu). Moreover, kaitiakitanga is a fundamental means by which survival is ensured – survival in spiritual, economic and political terms. (Kawharu, 2000, p 351)

Consequently, while the concept is most commonly associated with the care management and stewardship of natural resources, Kawharu clearly establishes that kaitiakitanga can also be considered more broadly in terms of care and stewardship functions in the human realm, within a societal context.

Discussion

This discussion presents three aspects of care ethics – care, justice and privileged irresponsibility; acknowledgement of past injustices; and how the embedded market philosophy in health and social care provision fails to appreciate, capture or adequately fund caring activities or tikanga.

Care, justice and privileged (ir)responsibility

Tronto (2013) and Barnes (2012a) surface privileged irresponsibility as a way in which power is actioned to maintain the status of particular peoples at the expense of others. People who inhabit positions of power, conventionally gendered and at the expense of marginalised groups, enable their power to continue. In order to inhabit a position of power, privilege benefits from care and support, but this is largely unacknowledged. Moreover, power sustained through care and support is likely to ensure that others are not provided with what they need in order to flourish, and therefore marginalisation, poverty and inequality are sustained. In the situation of colonised societies, the disparities are deep and entrenched as evidence of the processes of colonisation and its associated and continuing harms. As Tronto (2013, p 127) states:

The problem also is that those who have benefitted from past injustice have a great incentive to forget that fact, whether they perpetrated injustice or were simply bystanders who benefitted from the unjust acts of others, and those who have been so harmed cannot grasp how the world can go forward simply by ignoring or burying the past.

Interestingly, in Aotearoa/New Zealand, Borell et al (2009) identify that Māori are constructed as privileged in the dominant discourses of social life, as recipients of interventions aimed at ameliorating disparity, despite significant on-going disparities in wealth, health and education when compared to the settler community. The construct of privilege is consistent with the criticisms aimed at positive discrimination or positive action elsewhere, namely that certain privileges are offered to one group that are not offered to others without recourse to justice. Acknowledgements of past injustices resulting in the need for such positive action are conveniently forgotten, and instead claims are made about the lack of privilege available for the dominant group, in a bid to sustain such privileges that are 'invisible and unquestioned' (Borell et al, 2009, p 34).

Two key tenets of neoliberalism that have crept into aspects of everyday life are self-responsibility and life-style choice. Deprivations are explained away as life-style choices and a lack of self-responsibilisation. Borell et al (2009, p 44) note:

> More common understandings of health and social disparities continue to center around notions of individual responsibility, lifestyle choices and risk-taking behaviors. Such arguments deflect criticism and/or responsibility from those who do not suffer disadvantage and put the blame for disadvantage onto those who do.

Tronto and Barnes call for the recognition of privilege as the starting point for the acknowledgement of inequality and the power and position to be able to do something about ameliorating that imbalance. A just society would work toward the reduction of inequality as the key tenet of governmental intervention, and in colonised societies that justice would be determined by indigenous peoples.

Past injustices and the hurt and harms that continue today

Colonisation, justified as a global social movement that intended to improve the conditions of colonised people, assumed beneficence in terms of care that is now considered obsolete from a position of racial, cultural, religious and technological superiority (Walker, 1990). Many of the institutions and practices that justified the civilisation processes as 'care' continue to be present in colonised societies. Values and practices associated with colonisation are historically and politically located, but it would be wrong to suggest that we live in a world that is postcolonial, as the implications of colonisation are very much pertinent to the health and well-being of colonised people. Tronto (2013, p 24) notes that to define all attempts at care as good care would mean that 'to do so is to allow ourselves to be misled by the ways in which care can function discursively to obscure injustices'. These injustices may be past or current, but responses that are characterised by neoliberalism mean that any past injustices are ignored and no redress is permitted (Tronto, 2013, p 43).

Any cursory glance at how indigenous populations fare around the world indicates significant disadvantages in life expectancy, over-representation in prison and mental health populations, poorer health with higher incidence of preventable diseases, and poorer housing, income and education outcomes when compared with the dominant group. Health is the most often-cited disparity. The United Nations (2009, p 67) report states:

> Many illnesses that have a disproportionate impact on indigenous peoples, especially problems of mental health, are related to the colonialist and racist structures that cause indigenous communities to be some of the poorest and most marginalized in the world. Not only have indigenous peoples experienced a collective history of genocide, dispossession and dislocation, manifestations of these violent forces persist today …

So, to what extent does it matter to acknowledge past injustices, and in what ways do acknowledgements function to ease the trauma of colonisation? Acknowledgements have been made in the form of apology from governments to colonised people for specific traumas sanctioned by previous governments such as the 'Stolen Generation' in Australia (see Hage, 2000). While these are welcome, they do not carry the weight of responsibility and action beyond the specific trauma. It is necessary that past injustices are defined by indigenous populations to more broadly promote equality.

Embedded market philosophy fails caring activities or tikanga

Tronto (2013, p 38) has observed that neoliberalism fails those who, for one reason or another, are disenfranchised citizens of the state. Neoliberalism places significance on choice (particularly in consumption of goods or services), yet fails to recognise that, in the lived experience of many citizens, choice is denied through poverty, illiteracy, illness and or other forms of marginalisation. Choice for these citizens is not an option. In the Aotearoa/New Zealand context the Treaty of Waitangi ostensibly ensures that Māori have rights to live as Māori and in accordance with Māori customs and values, *and* to enjoy the privileges and rights extended to any other citizen. In reality, socioeconomic disparity as a consequence of past injustices and harms, coupled with the desire to uphold Māori world-views, philosophies, values and practices can, at best, clash with a neoliberal agenda and, at worst, result in pockets of the Māori populations becoming even more marginalised.

One such example where the neoliberal agenda completely fails an indigenous world-view is in the area of health and social care. Tronto, citing McClusky (2003, p 816), observes that neoliberalism 'confers superior citizenship status on those centrally identified with the market – they are members of the public whose gains count' Tronto (2013, p 40). For Māori, caring for those who are infirm, unwell, aged or otherwise disadvantaged has less to do with providing a cost-effective service as rational actors in the care marketplace and more to do with the concepts of whanaungatanga, manaakitanga and kaitiakitanga. Wholehearted and unquestioning support of this agenda by successive governments has not only led to the usurping of these core values, but to their corruption whereby the market now attempts to 'purchase' these concepts in health and social service contracts as it would purchase bedpans and counselling hours. Ironically, while recognising the utility of these values to improving care outcomes, the market fails to appreciate, capture or adequately fund these culturally motivated caring activities. Thus, in mental health service provision, delivering a culturally appropriate service places additional obligations and responsibilities on the provider; responsibilities which are not recognised in the contracts for service through remunerating either the additional work undertaken or the additional skills and expertise required to undertake the work in a culturally safe manner (Boulton, 2007). This failure of the neoliberal agenda to recognise anything other than the supremacy of the market has resulted in what commentators have termed 'Māori resistance'. As Bargh (2007, p 15) explains,

> The threat that neoliberal practices pose for indigenous way of life, most importantly by extending the market mechanism to all areas of life previously governed in other ways, is the reason for much of Māori resistance. The extension of the market mechanism seeks to override the ways that Māori have previously thought about and

governed their lives and resources. Neoliberal policies threaten Māori world-views, which understand the relationship between Māori and resources as diverse and holistic, rather than market-based. For many Māori, if neoliberal ways of thinking cannot coexist alongside other world-views, but instead seek to dominate and colonise Māori world-views, then these practices must be resisted.

Conclusion: inhabiting the moral boundary

An intentional shift away from recolonising practices led us to ask whether care ethics, in its challenge to neoliberalism, could be supported and informed by indigenous knowledges. We selected three concepts that are interwoven and connected and that resound widely in indigeneity. They support our view that indigenous knowledge can inform the habitat of care ethics. Indigenous cultures have a long tradition of species activities of maintaining and sustaining the world that includes relationships with the past and responsibilities to the future. Guardians of the land may be human, but they may also be rocks, trees and mountains and this has a specific impact on the framing and understanding of environmental concerns such as fracking or deep sea drilling – it is not only the extraction of the minerals from the land that is of concern, but it may also be that elements of the environment are moved, that sea creatures are disturbed and that traditional fishing and resource rights are disrupted or lost. Tronto (2013, p 52) discusses responsibility extending beyond the human realm within 'some form of relation – presence, biological, historical, or institutional ties; or some other form of "interaction"' (p 53). Indigenous peoples are unable to achieve or maintain well-being without the required connection to the land and each other.

Care operates as a species activity, where work and care are balanced, such as responsibilities, obligations and contributions in terms of time and money to care for resources and institutions of culture, such as waahi tapu (sacred sites) and marae (meeting places). This echoes the care ethic view of recognition of the need for collective effort for care of the collective, in order to create time to work and care (Tronto, 2013, pp 87–8). Collective interdependence remains an expectation in indigenous cultures, where societal responsibility structures and governs relationships, or how we may consider caring citizens.

Indigenous political processes are often consensual, where each member who is affected by the issue under discussion has the right to a voice or to direct representation within the iwi if they choose. Care and politics are intertwined rather than divorced into separate spheres. In Aotearoa, the requirement that tribal leaders make informed decisions on behalf of the whole tribe and that such decisions arise from tribal consensus results in what some consider unduly protracted Treaty of Waitangi settlement processes. However, tribal leaders recognise that, in having the mandate of the people, decisions are made today for the benefit of the whole tribe, rather than individuals within it, and for future generations yet to come. This often prompts conflicts in Pākeha governance processes (Jackson, 2010).

In 1993 Tronto set out three moral boundaries, and her more recent work seeks to transform politics through recognition of the need for care as a central concept in everyday lives and actions. Ethics of care questions the moral boundaries that sustain prevalent structural and intersectional inequalities (Tronto, 1993). Morality and politics are not separate, and Tronto argues that care can serve as the moral value and political achievement of a good society. In relation to achieving justice for people who experience inequalities, care as a value and a political achievement enables questioning the morality of political action that sustains oppression. Seeking answers to why and how oppression is accepted in certain circumstances surfaces a conversation that is currently framed very differently. Indigenous peoples' struggle for recognition and self-determination is based on different world-views that value interdependence and collective care and that are procedurally situated and complex. The moral boundary is inhabited with established values and practices that breathe life into care ethics.

Note

[1]   From an estimated 100,000 in the late 18th century (Te Ara: The Encyclopedia of New Zealand), the population dropped to 32,000 at the turn of the 20th century, and has grown to 560,000 in the 2013 census.

SEVEN

Privilege and responsibility in the South African context

Vivienne Bozalek

Introduction

This chapter has as its goal a focus on recognising how, both historically and currently, *privilege, responsibility* and *privileged irresponsibility*, all central notions of the political ethics of care, can be used to understand political, economic and cultural issues in the South African context. Although the chapter focuses on the South African context in particular, the understandings generated by an analysis of privileged irresponsibility with respect to the politics of gender, race, generation and class can easily be applied to other geopolitical contexts. The chapter is divided into three main parts. The first section focuses on the notions of privilege, responsibility and privileged irresponsibility and examines how it is possible to maintain privilege and privileged irresponsibility, using Plumwood's (1993; 2002) notion of dualisms. The second section provides South African examples of how privileged irresponsibility can be used to analyse historical and current power dynamics across race, class and gender by focusing on the social work curriculum. The third part of the chapter looks at how it is possible to act on privileged irresponsibility, by examining some South African examples of this. The discussion and conclusion provide some recommendations of how privileged irresponsibility may be addressed.

Privilege, responsibility and privileged irresponsibility

Privilege has been defined by various authors as unearned social and structural advantages which benefit dominant groups or those who occupy positions of power in society, at the expense of marginalised groups (McIntosh, 2010; Pease, 2010, 2011; Wiggan, 2011; Sensoy and DiAngelo, 2012). These conditions are generally taken for granted, invisible and normalised in society, and privilege is thus an unmarked status, rarely recognised, particularly by those who benefit from it. The advantages which the privileged have access to are actually those which should be enjoyed by all parties, as they would be in a just society, but which are restricted to those with a dominant status in unequal societies (Tronto, 1993; Schiele, 1996; Swigonski, 1996; Hardy, 2001; Sullivan, 2006; McIntosh, 2010; Pease, 2010; Wiggan, 2011; Sensoy and DiAngelo, 2012; Sholock, 2012).

As Swigonski (1996) notes, privileges make people feel at home in the world and take for granted that they are the centre of their world where social, political, economic and other resources are available. Exclusion, on the other hand, de-centres or marginalises individuals who have less access to such resources. Moreover, those who are marginalised are commonly deprived of the discursive space to define themselves in their own terms and have, therefore, to subscribe to the definitions of themselves by those who are in power in order to survive. Asante's (1988) concept of 'loss of terms', a metaphor for Africa's economic and social relationships to the Western world, is a useful one here, as it refers to the physical and mental aggression to which Africans were subjected, thereby being moved off their physical, social, mental and economic terms by the Western world (Swigonski, 1996, p 157). Asante (1988) refers to European slave drivers as moving Africans off their physical terms, missionaries as moving Africans off their religious terms and capitalists as moving Africans off their economic terms.

Generally, those who occupy privileged positions are not as aware of the distinctiveness of their beliefs and practices as those who are in less powerful positions, because the privileged practices are regarded by all as being self-evident and 'normal' and therefore exempt from scrutiny. The idea that whites do not have a culture is mirrored in many white people's own unconsciousness of being raced (Frankenberg, 1993) and in their engaging in cultural practices that are unmarked and unnamed. Frankenberg (1993) posits that part of the work of whiteness is the generation of norms so that white beliefs seem universal, natural and timeless, thus invisible and not socially and politically constructed. As a result of this, the white western self has remained largely unexamined.

Responsibility, on the other hand, is seen from a political ethics of care perspective as the willingness to act in order to do something about identified needs in society, it also requires acknowledgement that we are implicated in social conditions and structural injustices (Tronto, 1993; 2013). Stephen Esquith (2010, p 27) believes that responsibility involves those who have benefited from the 'suffering of heterogeneous subaltern populations at the hands of severe violence', in which he includes hunger, poverty, wars, genocide and pandemics. He sees the necessity of 'correcting the myopic self-understanding' of those who have benefited in this way (Esquith, 2010, p 27). Margaret Walker (2006) regards it as necessary to leverage responsibility for systemic oppression by moving people to a fuller understanding of how they may be related to it. Young (2011), on the other hand, does not think that we should direct liability to certain groups of people, but views all parties – both the privileged and the disadvantaged – as being implicated in structural injustices, and promotes a shared connected model of responsibility.

Following from these views of privilege and responsibility, privileged irresponsibility was a concept developed by Joan Tronto through the course of her academic writing career (see Bozalek, 2014 for a more elaborated description of the history of privileged irresponsibility). In her latest work on democracy and caring, Tronto (2013) describes privileged irresponsibility as those (privileged groups) who get a 'pass' out of responsibility by justifying why they should not be doing such work. In dominant discourses of contemporary society, the work ethic reigns supreme and care is not generally acknowledged as a valuable social activity or as proper work. Those who occupy positions of power have an interest in having their needs met without acknowledging that they are able to function because of the care they receive from others (Tronto, 2013). Furthermore, they tend, from a position of privileged irresponsibility, to ignore the needs of those who are doing the hands-on care-giving work for them.

From the lens of a political ethics of care, one cannot assume that the world consists of independent, self-sufficient, equally placed humans – we are all dependent at different times of our lives, and dependents all need to be cared for (Tronto, 1993, 2013; Sevenhuijsen, 1998; Kittay, 1999; Robinson, 1999, 2011; Olthuis, Kohlen and Heier, 2014). In terms of the ethics of care, dependency is seen as a normal part of human life, and one which should be considered in social sharing of burdens, just as education, health services and road maintenance are (Kittay, 2002a). Recognition of the centrality of care is contradicted by the common assumption that care should be a familial obligation only, rather than a social and public responsibility. This societal devaluing of care is important to consider in terms of the responsibilities that family members assume, as well as the underpaid forms of employment (largely domestic work) that many black South African women have been obliged to pursue as their only means of survival.

The feminist philosopher Val Plumwood's (1993, 2002) concept of dualism and its associated properties provides a useful analysis of how privileged irresponsibility has been maintained in the South African context. By dualism Plumwood means the way in which people are othered or misrecognised by being devalued. Plumwood (1993, 2002) insightfully identifies a number of means by which a hierarchical dualised relationship to the other is created. These characteristics include the following.

- Backgrounding – by this Plumwood means the denial of dependency on a subordinated other, where the services of the other are used but this contribution is not acknowledged or is backgrounded. This mechanism of dualism is the closest to Tronto's (1993; 2013) notion of privileged irresponsibility, where those in a position of racial/gendered privilege benefit from and make use of the services of the other, who meets their needs. Those privileged by racial, class or gendered markers neither recognise nor take responsibility for their own privileges or the other's lack of such privileges. Both Plumwood and Tronto hypothesise that it is fear of being dependent on the other and of acknowledging dependencies that creates this obfuscation of the value of the contribution that the other makes.
- Radical exclusion – this is where the privileged group make sure that there is a maximisation of separation between themselves and the marginalised group in order to disassociate from and thereby mark the other as a lower or inferior being. Unbridgeable separation is achieved by magnifying the degraded differential activities or qualities ascribed to the other. This process ensures that no continuities or similarities are perceived, thus no identification with the other can occur. Such a polarisation sets up a perceived (but false) dichotomy and naturalises domination by portraying denigrated qualities as inherent in the other. An example of different spheres is the public and private realms, which are seen as two worlds that operate separately and have nothing in common. Physical distance – as in the separated geographical areas created through forcible removals during and before the apartheid regime in South Africa – serves to maximise differences and maintain hyperseparation between the privileged and the marginalised groups.
- Incorporation – here the other is defined as a lack, a negation or an absence, and is recognised only in relation to the self or the master's desires or needs. Because the other is negated and seen as having none of the desirable qualities, there is no space for them and they are colonised, subsumed or incorporated into the master. This leads to the fourth characteristic.
- Instrumentalism – by being defined only as a means to someone else's ends the other is regarded as an instrument and so objectified. The other, having no intrinsic value, falls outside moral consideration and

is regarded as a resource for the more important one. Identities such as 'good girl' or 'good wife' are constructed instrumentally rather than morally, as, in themselves, they fall outside moral consideration.

• Homogenisation – differences that exist, like the multiplicity of languages, between those who are inferiorised, are regarded as being unimportant, denied or undermined and belittled, as they are not regarded to be of any importance. Homogenisation thus produces binarisms, dividing the world into two perspectives – that of the master and that of the other. The important view is that of the master, not that of the other. The other is not regarded in a personal or unique way, as an individual, but as an interchangeable resource to serve the master's needs. The privileged and marginalised groups are also regarded as very different from each other, which justifies the unequal treatment that they receive.

Instances of privileged irresponsibility from the South African context

As the Australian social work educator Bob Pease (2011, p 410) notes, '[s]ocial work education provides an excellent opportunity for all students to interrogate their privilege and unearned entitlements critically within social divisions, whether these divisions are related to gender, class, race, sexuality, or other forms of privilege'.

At the University of the Western Cape (UWC) (a historically black or disadvantaged university in South Africa), black working–class South African social work students conducted a Family in Community assignment between their second and third years of study in the social work curriculum, where they reported on family practices. The students were given questions about how race, class and gender had impacted on their family members and themselves (see Bozalek, 2010, 2012 for further details on this), and in these assignments it became evident that many instances of privileged irresponsibility were recorded.

Some students regarded the whole colonial enterprise, traced from the Dutch settlers, as purposefully having set out to separate family members by making life extremely difficult in rural areas through the imposition of hut taxes and the monetarisation of relationships. Historically, the conquest of land by white settlers made it possible for whites to make use of blacks as cheap labour for the mines and farms and as domestic workers to maintain white households. Family members were prevented from being together, through legislation that sought to control the movement of those marked black: it restricted those who were not useful for fulfilling white needs from being in urban areas, and allowed others access to urban areas in order to fulfil these needs. Those marked as black were moved around to service the needs of those marked as white, thus reinforcing privileged irresponsibility on the part of the white population. That only certain family members were regarded as useful for these purposes, while others were redundant, had the effect of separating members from each other, thus affecting the forms of human association considered important for human well-being or flourishing.

In what Glen Elder (2003, p 13) has referred to as the 'procreational geography of apartheid', poverty compelled men from rural areas to seek work as migrants, but women and children were not permitted to join their husbands. In shaping the lives of black men, women and children differently, apartheid can be regarded as not only a racist, but also a sexist and ageist body of social policies, which had diverse implications for students' family members, depending on their gendered and generational status. Several students viewed their fathers' absences as being problematic in that it led to family members becoming estranged from each other, with men failing to give reliable and consistent financial support to distant children and wives, having children with other women and sometimes failing to maintain contact with their family members, or even to see them again.

Students' accounts also indicated that the denigration of family members in their paid employment as domestic workers, for example, had repercussions not only for the person directly employed in terms of their views of themselves as inferior relative to their employers, but for members of their families too, who were also trained to regard themselves and their family practices as inferior.

In South Africa, through othering and inferiorising Africans into homogenised categories of 'maids and factotums', whites were assured that an extended population, designated specifically to provide services for them and meet their everyday needs, would be available – this was the case in the past and is still largely the prevalent position in South Africa. Domestic workers in South Africa continue to be a vulnerable group of people in relation to care giving, as Shireen Ally (2009) has indicated. Thus, through being categorised as maids and factotums, Africans as others can be seen as objectified and regarded only as instruments to fulfil white needs.

The African-American feminist writer Barbara Omolade (1994) has described how white women and men in the US were able to pursue careers outside the home because they were buttressed by black women who maintained white middle-class households by caring for their bodily needs. The same applies very clearly in South Africa, where there has long been a practice whereby poor black women provide cheap domestic service for even less for those whites who would not be considered wealthy (Cock, 1989; Le Roux, 1995; Ally, 2009). This practice has not been confined to whites employing black domestic workers, and now, as a significant black middle class is developing, the practice is increasingly being extended into their homes too. The process of instrumentalism of those relegated to this kind of work has meant that no regard is given to the personal circumstances of black women domestic workers or to the needs they or their own family members may have.

What was evident in the students' accounts was how othering of students' mothers, grandmothers and other female relatives has led to privileged irresponsibility in care provision. Students' mothers, aunts and grandmothers took care of people in households other than their own, and for minimal wages, while their own children had no access to them (Le Roux, 1995). The consequences of live-in domestic work for the family relationships of the domestic worker can be seen as a form of privileged irresponsibility in that the needs of the privileged were serviced at the expense of those who were marginalised; secondly, there are the consequences of migrant work in taking people away from their close-kin relatives, where other female relatives were obliged to do the care-giving work of the dependent relatives on an unpaid basis; thirdly, there are the consequences of forced relocation in separating previously cooperating and mutually supportive kin from one another.

The following is an excerpt from a student's family profile:

> My father was working as a slave in this farm. He was doing all the work, he was the garden boy [derogatory term which employers used for the men who did the garden for them], he was ploughing big fields alone, milking cows in the morning and in the evening and he had to spend the whole day in the field looking after the cattle, sheep, goats etc. At the age of 15 I was working as a domestic worker and that was very painful because the work was very hard for me, and what frustrated me worse was that I was never asked by my father's employers to work instead I was forced and I was told if I didn't want to work I had to leave that farm. What about my help at home for my sisters? Who was going to look after them? That was very painful. (Female rural African student, Family Profile 63)

The account above is a good example of the injustices that family members were subjected to in relation both to their paid employment and to their ability to give and receive care. It also reflects the extent to which resident farm workers' family members were regarded as sources of unpaid labour on the basis that the relationship between land-owner/farmer and working resident was one that required all members of the worker's household to provide labour power in exchange for the wage paid to the household head and the right to reside on farm land (Sharp and Spiegel, 1990). Both the student and her father were subjected to harsh labour conditions, with the father single-handedly having to engage in many different onerous tasks. The notion of privileged irresponsibility is starkly visible in this student's account, as the father is not recognised as an adult human being (the student describes his status as a garden 'boy'). His own needs for limits on the amount of work and for rest and adequate compensation were ignored. Furthermore, his dependency needs in relation to his family members were completely disregarded, with him being regarded rather as a head of a household that was understood to constitute a single labour-supplying unit (including his daughter) and whose sole purpose was to provide services to the employer. The coercion of the student to engage in domestic work for the employer at the threat of expulsion and at the expense of caring for her own siblings indicates the extent to which the needs of students and their family members were subsumed to the needs of those in privileged positions, in this instance, the employer and whoever resided in the employer's household. The exploitative and exclusionary practices with regard to paid employment placed many students and their family members in the painful predicament of being unable to attend to the needs of their dependents, both through their lack of time to spend with their dependents, and their lack of resources for meeting their needs.

Students also reported acts of privileged irresponsibility from a gendered perspective in their own households. They made observations corresponding to Tronto's (1993, 2013) notion of privileged irresponsibility, where they commented on how men took it for granted that their needs would be met, not considering how they were benefiting from women's work. Below is an example of a student who is conscious of her father's privileged irresponsibility (although she does not label it as such) with regard to care giving, and his obliviousness to the struggles of the woman as she attempts to cope with the multitude of tasks at hand.

I think that both men and women have to take care of their children, to give them love and care they deserve. It is very painful to watch a man sitting in the dining room reading a paper whilst the woman is in the kitchen cooking carrying a crying child on her back with others pulling her down with her dresses asking for food. In my opinion every household work has to be shared equally between men and women, boy and girls so as to live a harmonious life. (Family Profile 46)

How can privileged irresponsibility be addressed?

As has been observed in the section on privilege at the beginning of this chapter, the privileged tend to view their situations as 'normal' or 'natural'. According to the capabilities approach (Nussbaum, 1995, 2001; Sen, 1995, 2001), those who are in positions of privilege would generally not want to relinquish their advantages, which they may tend to take for granted, while those who are in positions of disadvantage may often not know of possibilities that would improve their situations. Long-established privilege or deprivation can lead, respectively, to high or low levels of desire (Sen, 1995). People's desires can therefore not be used as reliable indicators of justice. The capabilities approach thus does not see individual preferences as being reliable indicators of human needs, as those who are advantaged or disadvantaged easily become accustomed to their situations and adjust their expectations and aspirations accordingly. How, then, is it possible to resist privileged irresponsibility?

In looking at how these practices can be resisted, South African UWC social work students provided examples of practices in their families where gendered assumptions in relation to practices had been subverted. Alison Bailey, the American philosopher (2000), has described as 'traitorous' those subjects who belong to dominant groups yet resist the usual assumptions and practices of these groups. She distinguishes between 'privilege-cognisant' and 'privilege-evasive' white scripts in discussing race traitors. Privilege-cognisant whites (those who are conscious of and recognise their privileged position) refuse to engage in the 'daily collaboration of performances of historically pre-established scripts' (Bailey, 2000, p 296). On the other hand, privilege-evasive scripts (these are similar to what Joan Tronto (1993, 2013) has called being in a position of privileged irresponsibility) re-inscribe a racial order in which white lives are valued at the expense of the lives of people of colour. These ideas can be similarly used when considering the category of gender. A gender traitor or a privilege-cognisant man would try to understand the privileges granted to him and be critical of these, finding ways to develop alternative scripts.

As an illustration of the concept of gender traitor, I refer to the family profile of a Muslim woman student from a coloured township in Cape Town in which various privilege-cognisant scripts can be discerned in her brother's life history and then in the description of how he shared in household tasks. The brother has a critically reflective consciousness of his gendered behaviour. He values and acknowledges the positive side of rejecting his male script and being a gender traitor in his development of conflict resolution through debate rather than aggression. He is aware of himself as a member of a privileged group and is described by the student as initially resistant to giving up his privileges, but then relinquishing them and later willingly engaging in them as a result of pressure from his sisters and mother. As Alison Bailey (2000, p 296) comments, traitorousness involves breaking old habits and developing new ones. The father similarly engages in tasks that are the traditional domain of women. The student describes how he manages to resist even the dominant gendered script of the Islamic faith.Student's brother's life story:

> My sisters reckoned that I did not keep myself busy enough, and since my mother was adamant I was not to receive any special favours, I learnt to sweep, scrub and polish wooden floors, ironing and even mixing cake when Rashieda needed a strong arm. During winter I usually had to make a fire in a paraffin tin so we had hot coals to warm ourselves during the cold evenings.

Student's description of brother's role in household tasks:

> Zahied, under much protest at first, had to assist his sister in domestic chores, and later came to realise that there is no such thing as a completely women task or male task. He is even involved in babysitting his niece Nadia and nephew Monde (a task normally done by women competently). Basically I think it is up to the individual if he or she is so indoctrinated by stereotypical notions of what men's and women's roles in caring for other and domestic chores are, or are they willing to make that change?

These accounts of challenging gendered privileged irresponsibility on the part of family members can be regarded as examples of Foucault's (1982, p 785) notion of transformation, which requires not that we 'discover what we are' but, rather, that we 'refuse what we are'.

While there were instances of some students' being able to resist privileged irresponsibility, such as those described above, most students' accounts revealed how misrecognition was interiorised so that students and their family members colluded in their own subjugation, whether in terms of race, class, gender or generation. In Foucauldian terms, such interiorisation and conceding to the denigration of the values and practices of those who lack privileges, reflects the power of dominant discourses for the making of docile subjects. However, other accounts revealed how students and their family members maintained a critical stance towards the misrecognition they experienced, and that some were able to resist it, with some students reporting that they and their family members were able to identify and contest the authority of dominant norms. This is a significant step for students and their family members in being able to regain recognition of themselves as fully human and capable of participating with others as equals.

Discussion and conclusion

What lessons can be derived from the South African examples of privileged irresponsibility and of resistance to such privileged irresponsibility? The student accounts show how privileged groups have managed to maintain their advantages historically and currently in the South African context, through the exploitation and denigration of certain groups of people. There were also a few examples of how people managed to question their sense of entitlement through traitorous identities (Bailey, 2000) and act upon this. However, with regard to challenging privileged irresponsibility, given its ubiquitous nature across the markers of gender, race and class, its invisibility and the mechanisms of dualism that serve to bolster it, one may ask whether it is enough to hope that people will come to the realisation themselves and will act on it.

In order to act upon privileged irresponsibility, it would be necessary for all – those who benefit from privileges as well as those who are exploited and denigrated through the provision of their services – to become aware of Plumwood's (1993, 2002) mechanisms of dualism and how these serve to perpetuate the status quo.

I propose Iris Young's (2011) social connection model of responsibility as a way of addressing privileged irresponsibility. This model includes all parties in a shared responsibility for addressing privileges. It goes beyond merely listening and dialoguing with the other as is proposed by some in relation to privileged irresponsibility (see, for example, Sholock (2012), who proposes a methodology for the privileged the embraces the discomforts of epistemic uncertainty as a treasonous act, or Pease (2010), who suggests attentive listening and dialogical engagements across difference and inequality). Young (2011) distinguishes her social connection model from the liability model where particular agents are singled out as being guilty and are blamed and found liable for harms. Thus, responsibility for participating in structural processes that lead to unjust outcomes is shared. Here responsibility is regarded as forward looking, as it is on-going rather than backward looking, except to understand the relationships between policies and practices leading to outcomes. Young (2011) views responsibility as a political notion, which can be discharged through collective action.

In terms of addressing privileged irresponsibility in the curriculum, the notion that we are all implicated is also the basis of a pedagogy of discomfort, developed by Boler and Zembylas (2003) as a useful framework for understanding, teaching and learning about difference. This pedagogy invites students and lecturers to critique their deeply held assumptions, and to destabilise their views of themselves and their worlds, reconstruct previously held views and, by doing so, to move to new insights and dispositions (see Bozalek, Carolissen and Leibowitz, 2014). The 'discomfort' within this pedagogy impacts upon all members of a group, whether these are members of dominant or marginalised groups. A pedagogy of discomfort is therefore a more encompassing notion in that it is not just directed at those who are privileged, as all people are regarded as being implicated, and we are all subject to hegemonic discourses.

Since no one escapes hegemonic views, overcoming privileged irresponsibility will thus require all parties to 'refuse what we are' and act on this, rather than assuming that it is only a particular group that needs to do this.

EIGHT

Empathy in pursuit of a caring ethic in international development

Diego de Merich

Introduction: positioning development ethics after the Millennium Development Goals

The year 2015 will mark the conclusion of the Millennium Development Goals (MDGs). Met with great fanfare in international policy-making circles with the UN Millennium Declaration in 2000, the MDGs have sought to ameliorate the condition of countless poor around the world by focusing on attainable targets relating to their quality of life (broadly on health and disease, education, gender equality and the environment). For its part the UN General Assembly vowed to 'spare no effort' to promote 'respect for all internationally recognised human rights and fundamental freedoms, including the right to development' (UN, 2000, Sec V-24). This new policy framework found its normative justifications in the Human Capabilities Approach (HCA), an idea of justice that takes freedom and capabilities as central to its articulation of the good. In a development context, people are seen as 'shaping their own destiny, and not just as passive recipients of the fruits of cunning development plans' (Sen, 1999, p 53). Sen's articulation of freedom as the constitutive basis for well-being in *human* development[1] and the practical applications of this foundational premise that were realised through his association with Mahbub ul Haq[2] have made him the single leading justice theorist in the field of development ethics (Gasper and Truong, 2010, p 69).

At a structural level, however, critics of the MDGs raise the doubt that they have served only to depoliticise and compartmentalise aspects of human life and experience into discrete goals, thus ignoring the interconnectedness of many of those aspects with respect to inequality and deprivation. Reflecting a neoliberal logic that 'colonises' everyday practices and narrows recognition of these realities to discrete statistical measures, these goals and targets provide a 'superficial treatment of complex issues, and [abstract] them from structural inequalities and the specificities of place' (Wilson, 2014, p 6; see also Saith, 2006). Furthermore, these structures obfuscate relationships of care and caring that occur beneath (and despite) them. These *caringscapes* (McKie et al, 2002) constitute 'informal interdependencies across the lifecourse, at different spatial scales, [that] can be enacted through a variety of forms of communication, including expressive embodiment' (McEwan and Goodman, 2010, p 105). They resist discrete categorisation and speak to the foundation for a critical ethic of development; one that attends to vulnerability experienced by developing communities and the relationships of care that sustain them in the face of that vulnerability.

Indeed 'critical' development scholars Des Gasper and Trahn-Dam Truong suggest a deepened understanding of development that is based on four dimensions. In contrast to Sen's 'capabilities' approach or 'development as freedom', they weave together feminist care ethics, notions of human security and ideas of the Buddhist 'relational self' to describe these elements as follows:

- 'Development ethics should enrich its conception of the human being. Vulnerability and capability are two sides of the same coin' and care is what connects these two sides.
- 'Development ethics should enrich our notions of well-being'.
- An ethics of care could serve to reorient our understanding of moral responsibility, 'emphasizing both the interconnected nature of belonging and empathy as a basic human emotion'.
- It recognises 'the reality that human processes, and persons, have escaped from national containers' (see Tronto, Chapter Two in this volume) and requires 'an end to the perceptual and therefore moral blindness regarding interstate care provision'. (Gasper and Truong, 2010, p 89)

Care ethics provides a rich field of critical inquiry from which a development theorist might draw insight. Whether articulations of care in the context of globalisation (Hankivsky, 2006), international relations, development and human security (Robinson, 1999; 2006; 2011); to cosmopolitan theory (Clark Miller, 2010), to political theory, broadly conceived (Tronto, 1993; 2007; 2013; Hankivsky, 2004); whether in relation to virtue ethics (Slote, 2007), concepts of citizenship (Sevenhuijsen, 1998), institutions (Tronto, 2010) or natural law theory (Engster, 2007); or as a moral philosophy separate from purely virtue-based approaches (Held, 2006) or in parallel to Confucian thought (Li, 2008), care ethics intimates at the possibility of constructing an ethical framework for international development that is more open to the possibility of alternate visions of 'the good life'.[3] And yet, despite such critical insight into the nature of responsibility, empathy has never figured prominently in care theory. To date, Michael Slote (2007) is the only care theorist who puts the complex notion of empathy at the heart of his understanding of care. The purpose of this chapter is to examine the role that empathy and empathic learning play as the motivators for caring practices and responses to the perceived vulnerability of others. In highlighting the deontological approach Slote employs, I suggest that it misses the more transformative potentials of an ethics of care that seeks instead to find moral insight from empathic intersubjectivity. I then explore two programmes that reflect two styles of empathic learning. The first is the use of *immersions* in development settings. The second, the International Child Development Programme (ICDP), is only tangentially related to development 'proper', but, given its presence in over 27 countries and direct support by UNICEF, it can certainly be said to fall under the broader human development approach.[4] I seek to argue that if caring *practices* are meant to be responsive to the needs of care receivers, if attentiveness is one of the primary examples of ethical practice for care theorists, then empathy provides *a* method in answer to the questions of attentiveness 'to whom' or attentiveness 'how'.

Empathy: the epistemic bridge at the intersections of care

In his *The Ethics of Care and Empathy* (2007), Michael Slote takes a significant departure from earlier care ethicists with regard to how 'all-encompassing' a moral framework of 'care' and 'caring' should be considered. For him, it is from the earliest work on an *ethics* of caring – Nel Noddings' *Caring: A Feminine Approach to Ethics and Moral Education* – that a very common and perhaps ambiguously parochial understanding of care arose. According to Noddings, our most basic moral relations with people whom we have never met can never properly be subsumed under a morality of caring (which requires at least a modicum of temporal or spatial proximity). On questions of 'distant others', an ethic of traditional justice would have to prevail (see Barnes, Chapter Three in this volume). As a result of this basic distinction, most care theorists have since held care as being complementary to traditional justice/moral theory (Crittenden, 2001; Hankivsky, 2004; Held, 2006). In our greater understanding of human morality, therefore, care has been seen as most relevant to certain moral spheres but not to others. Slote, however, highlights the foundational role that empathy plays in any moral theory pertaining to care; care is then understood as a direct alternative to justice, whereby it can be used to understand all personal and political issues of morality and, more importantly, for the political action which would follow. For Slote, 'all, or almost all, the moral distinctions we intuitively or commonsensically want to make can be understood in terms of – or at least correlated with distinctions of empathy' (Slote, 2007, p 4). Furthermore, as was largely anticipated by moral sentimentalists of the Scottish Enlightenment, increasingly our knowledge of brain chemistry and psycho-social development is demonstrating that empathy is the primary mechanism involved in responses of caring, compassion and benevolence (see Baron–Cohen, 2011).

One clear distinction that is often made between care and justice theories is the former's rejection of deontological, Kantian or Categorical Imperative justifications for moral reasoning. Here, Slote seeks to differentiate himself from such a rejection. It is worth reviewing his elaboration of empathy before proposing another. For him, deontology is not 'a matter of principles or rules or rational considerations that oppose sentiments, but rather arises from, or can be understood in terms of, the sentiments themselves' (Slote, 2007, p 45). Rather than viewing deontological imperatives as extraneous principles or rules, from a care-theoretical standpoint, they can be justified on intuitive grounds – intuition or sentiment, itself, being one of the foundations of care ethics. Deontology is seen here as less 'categorical' and more contextual because, while agreement can be found that 'killing one to save five is morally wrong' at first glance, sentimental proximity to the individuals involved necessarily influences the decision or action taken. In other words, recognition of the empathic foundation of an intuitive moral reasoning helps to clarify where and how that categorical imperative may be less categorical.

Using David Wiggins' reading of Hume (Wiggins, 1991), Slote goes on to outline a 'thick' normativity that rests on Kant's distinction between categorical and hypothetical imperatives. Similar to the distinction between perfect and imperfect obligations, the argument can be described as follows: a person to whom a hypothetical claim is being made can fail to respond to that claim for want of desire or motive; a person to whom a categorical claim is being made cannot, lest she face moral criticism. However, he says, 'according to care ethics, it is or can be wrong for me not to help, say, my daughter, even if I have no desire to help her' (Slote, 2007, p 107). Furthermore, since Kant's description of these imperatives was to ground them in our everyday practices and understanding of morality, it is not inconceivable (according to Wiggins and Slote) that Hume had an *implicit* understanding of this distinction even if Kant was the first to explicitly articulate it. In other words, in his 'daughter' example, Slote finds a moral sentimentalist (care ethics) example of a Kantian categorical imperative. As it involves my own daughter, I would be morally criticised for not helping her and so, therefore, despite my lack of desire or motivation, I *must* (morally) help her.

Unfortunately this line of reasoning does two things. Firstly, it suggests an understanding of care ethics that is of the virtue ethics tradition (that care is primarily about a *disposition* to care, and most especially for familial relations). In so doing, secondly, it further reifies the nuanced distinction between proximate relationships of care and distant ones. Oddly, he makes an argument for deontology and categorical imperatives as an abstract justification for a 'thick' normativity within care-ethics sentimentalism, using the example of a relation that intuitively we would expect to be governed by emotion and, therefore, by concern *and* motivation. 'Of course' we would morally criticise this (somewhat difficult to imagine) father who has *no* desire to help his daughter. Yet it seems a rather 'thin' justification for this more 'thick' normative claim. Can this be the only example upon which to suggest that moral categorical imperatives (might) exist even within care-ethics sentimentalism? Slote's normative claims are predicated upon a virtue ethics understanding of care. I am, however, more inclined to agree with Virginia Held's understanding that while it may find its precursors in virtue ethics or moral sentimentalism, care ethics concerns itself primarily with caring *relations* (Held, 2006). Such relations capture not only the moral dispositions of the persons held in relation to one another, but also the objective results of caring (*responsiveness to* a stated or perceived need for example).

I suggest, however, that we might still maintain the centrality that Slote places on the role of empathy in care, but that we might do so without the need to bring our moral understanding of care back within the Kantian fold. If both empathy *and* care are understood as process and practice, respectively – the first a process of understanding or learning based on affect *and* cognition and the second a practice of commitment and responsiveness to an 'other' whom we stand in relation to – then it seems that the 'thin' understanding of normativity, described above, would suffice. If empathy is a *learning* process that highlights attentiveness to – emotional engagement with a situated responsiveness to an articulated need or vulnerability – then it is a better understanding of empathy that should be the focus of our normative evaluations. Furthermore, if caring practices are meant to be understood as *care full* – reflective of the view of the care receiver (Barnes, 2012a, p 74) – such empathic learning is central.

Empathy as intersubjective process

To instead understand empathy as a process of intersubjectivity and affective *cognition*, Louis Agosta's work (1984; 2010), James Marcia's (1987) and Michael Morrell's (2010) are helpful. As Marcia defines it, empathy 'requires an attitude or a stance of openness to another's experience' (Marcia, 1987, p 83). Describing the four aspects of empathy outlined by Theodore Reik in 1949, he shows that the process itself is guided by *identification, incorporation, reverberation* and *detachment*. Broadly speaking, these four steps involve contemplation of another person; internalising the other's experience; 'experiencing the other's experience while simultaneously attending to one's own cognitive and affective associations to that experience' (Marcia, 1987, p 83); moving away from that inner merging of self and other's emotional experience so as to be able to respond or act, fully cognisant of that separateness.

According to Agosta, the effect on the self is one of the defining results of this process. There are three ways, he argues, by which empathy leads to an enriched self:

> First, in relation to other individuals regarded collectively as an intersubjective community, empathy is part of the foundation of that intersubjectivity [...] Second, in relation to particular individuals, empathy furnishes a way of access to the other person's emotional life and of disclosing how our lives overlap and diverge. *Here the self is enriched by discovering the variety and multiplicity of experiences of which other individuals are capable.* Third, in the relation of the self to itself, empathy *entails an appreciation of how others are affected by oneself.* (Agosta, 1984, p 60; emphasis added)

What is striking about this description of empathy as a process that feeds, and is in turn fed by, intersubjectivity is that it implies an epistemology that is experiential and inherently social. The more we understand of others, the more we understand ourselves. Within the context of development studies, I contend that the implication is far reaching. As puerile as the logic might seem, the argument could then be made that an individual in a so-called developed country, in somehow participating in this empathic loop (empathy–intersubjectivity–empathy) or circuit, would understand not only the lived needs of some other but also how the self may have bearing on those needs. Equally possible is for that same person to simply re-evaluate her own understanding of 'need'. International development could no longer be seen as having a beginning (direct capital investment in infrastructure), a middle (International Monetary Fund structural adjustment policies) and an end (realisation of the MDGs). Rather, development – properly conceived as human development – will require a new appraisal of self and other as inherently intertwined. Under-development can be understood only in relation to over-development, with some equilibrium as the constant (negotiated, ruptured, fought over) goal.

In a similar vein, the strength of Michael Morrell's argument stems from his attempt at viewing various strands and definitions of empathy as parts of a multi-dimensional whole. While it's true that empathy involves emotion to a greater or lesser degree, this emotion is almost always invariably conditioned by, prompted by or the result of cognitive or rational processes (Morrell, 2010, p 61). Developing Mark Davis's 'organizational model of Empathy', Morrell describes a *process model of empathy* that includes *noncognitive* (primary circular reaction, motor mimicry), *simple cognitive* (direct association or labelling) and *advanced cognitive* (language-mediated associations or role-taking) processes (Morrell, 2010, p 64). These processes then interact with a number of other factors within the social functioning or performance of empathy (including an individual's biological capacities, the resultant social behaviour, the empathic concern engendered and so on). This entire complex is Morrell's 'process model', understanding empathy as a multi-dimensional construct.

Empathy in action: from immersions to the International Child Development Programme

Within the context of development programmes, 'immersions' have become a method by which development practitioners or government officials are brought into contact with the lived experiences of individuals or families in the developing world. It is believed that in this way the voices and perspectives of the poor will be better 'heard and integrated into new policy approaches and practices at a senior level' (IDS, 2004, p 3). Often a middle- or senior-level bureaucrat will be sent to a development context to speak with a family or to 'live' there for a day, a weekend or a week. Such an experience, it is thought, then informs future judgements and proposals made by the official, along with relayed accounts of lived experiences of the individuals that a programme may affect. As Carolyn Pedwell argues, these 'affective journeys' are understood as vehicles for self-transformation that then might 'contain the seeds of wider social and political transformation' (Pedwell, 2012, p 170).[5] As learners and guests, participating in the daily life and experiences of the focused subjects of development policy, practitioners are thought to take away more than basic learning or insight. These encounters 'challenge values and beliefs, and raise questions about the sort of people we are and want to be, and what we *do*' (Chambers, 2005, p 181).

Of course there is no simple template by which these immersions operate, nor are they necessarily more than a one-off interaction within the larger process of an organisation's development activities. Often they are guided by a particular theme or line of enquiry, sometimes they are unplanned or unexpected visits. The benefits of an average immersion, in addition to the sense of 'accountability' they engender, include: project monitoring, familiarisation with a new post, experiential realism, capacity building and programme development (Chambers, 2005, p 11). The key argument to be made here, however, is that such 'events' run the risk of being discrete activities, another in a series of boxes to be checked before the policy process continues apace. To use the theoretical distinctions highlighted above, they might be considered specific moments of empathic affect, rather than empathic processes maintained over time *within* the community in question. In comparison to programmes that instead deal with empathic learning directly within developing contexts (for the *sole purpose* of empathic awareness), these immersions, therefore, might better be described as 'sticking a toe in the shallow end of a pool'. They also fail to consider (explicitly) how vulnerability affects a care receiver's ability to even reflect upon or communicate her understanding of her situation, her needs or the response she may wish for.

> Extreme poverty and social exclusion humiliate people, cause them to lose confidence, and barricade them into silence. Their relationships with others are stifled. When people lose the strength to protest their reality, or when they know that their words are unwanted by others, silence can become a leaden weight on their hearts. Compounding the weight of silence, people know that even the right to free speech is not enough. (Skelton, 2014, p 72)

The work of the International Child Development Programme (ICDP) might be seen as providing a deeper expression for empathic engagement. Founded in 1992 in Norway, the ICDP runs projects in over 20 countries, including Tanzania, Mozambique, Colombia, Guatemala and Malaysia. It is important to emphasise that it is a programme that can (and does) operate in developed and developing contexts alike.[6] It is based on the idea that 'human beings are by nature social and that also means that we, as human beings, are particularly vulnerable in our social relationships because that is the domain of our suffering and our happiness' (ICDP, 2010, p 2). The broadly based educational programme, though aimed primarily at children and their care givers in local communities, is seen to have application in all other relationships of care (older people, youth, adults). The mandate (and even motto) of the organisation is a simple one: 'Empathy in Action'.

The main focus on 'empathy in action' is understood to be transferable across cultures and continents, 'based on recent research in child development that sensitises and enriches the relationship between caregivers and their children' (ICDP, 2008, p 1). It is important to stress that the only full, mixed-methods study into the effectiveness of the programme was conducted in 2009 by a group of academics from Norway and the UK. So as to factor in different emotional and cultural backgrounds, sample survey data was collected from the general population of participants, from members of ethnic minorities and from incarcerated fathers, all of whom attended basic ICDP training. In response to the basic question 'What is the impact of the programme on caregivers and caregiver-child relationships?' 82.6% noted some form of self-transformation and 55.6% noted change in the family (for example, caregiver–child relationship) (Sherr et al, 2011, p 99). Of considerable note, in terms of the 'environments' of recognition and care, it was interesting to participants in the incarcerated fathers group that after participation in the programme it was more likely that fathers would sit in the common room and chat with one another about their children; that in subsequent weeks even relations between inmates and prison staff were less combative (Sherr et al, 2011, p 75). In immigrant communities, of most note was the marked increase in improvement of self-perception felt on the part of mothers (Sherr et al, 2011, p 55). One recommendation of the report was to suggest more outreach to male parents in these communities.

While no such comprehensive survey study was conducted in the other countries (especially in the developing world) where the ICDP has been launched effectively, participant and trainer feedback all point, anecdotally, to very similar, positive outcomes. Parents experience what might be described as a self-transformation that qualitatively appears to result in more self-confidence in terms of parenting skills and ability, more affective connection between fathers and children, and overall more happy, peaceful relations between children or care receivers and care givers. A father in Guatemala who participated in the training commented:

> 'I have experienced something I never had as a child which is to be appreciated only because I am a person; this is what we need in our community and these guidelines in the booklet I received need to reach not only families and children *but also the elderly* in our community as they need it just as much.' (ICDP, 2009, p 9; emphasis added)

Trust is engendered by care givers' being able to share experiences and learn from one another how best to recognise vulnerability in a concrete 'other'. This ability to see oneself as nested within an array of caring relationships (from the familial to the international), then, constitutes the basis for a co-responsibility to action.

The introduction of 'immersions', I contend, represents a 'shallow' introduction to empathic understanding. The work of the ICDP, instead, is presented as a 'deep' application of empathic processes within both 'developed' *and* 'developing' communities. I have sought to structure a discussion of empathy that differentiates between its content (double representation)[7] as well as its process (affective-cognitive). This process, in turn, when added to previous theories about relational and care-ethical solutions to global development problems, leads to a deeper reflection on and understanding of a particular problem and suggests that a solution for care may not be the same in every 'centre' or context of care. The ICDP is not a development programme in the strictest sense. Rather than emphasising individual agency, as a rights-justice ethical approach might, it understands agency, dignity and self-worth as necessarily bound by the social contexts in which we find ourselves.

Conclusions

In attempting to suggest the centrality of empathy to our understanding of care ethics, I first addressed the 'Copernican revolution' claimed by Michael Slote – a paradigm shift which, by recognising empathy at the centre of all our relations, would change the nature of how we perceive moral philosophical questions, and then also how we practise care. Slote's narrower understanding of care ethics as falling squarely within the rubric of virtue ethics (care as disposition and not as relation) is combined with a Kantian deontology to be 'tacked onto' this central role for care ethics, ostensibly so as to provide a 'thick' normative basis for his claims. I reject both ideas (care as virtue and the very need for a 'thick' or Kantian normative basis for care ethics). In fact, the value argument is turned on its head here. By outlining the complex nature of empathy as process, the 'thick' philosophical underpinning of care comes from a stronger elaboration of the empathic learning practices that lead us to take moral or ethical decisions.

There are a number of ways by which an empathic approach to international development complements and builds upon recent literature on care, responsibility and empowerment within the fields of international relations (Robinson, 1999), post-development thought (Escobar, 2001) and political geography (Raghuram, Madge and Naxolo, 2009). Complementarity is found in a relational understanding of the nature of the problems at hand and of the actors involved in addressing those problems. It is within those relationships, problematic both spatially and temporally, that motivation to respond and to take responsibility is ultimately located. But specifically on the question of motivation to act, a recognition of the centrality of empathy to 'care full' practices of responsibility toward care receivers – and in recognising care receivers (in a development context) as care givers in their own right – it is possible to imagine an intersubjective mode of collective learning in international development that informs caring practices. Yes, care is embodied in existent practices across different spaces. But in encountering a care receiver (as in an immersion encounter), one focus of the practitioner should be on the caring relations within which the host family find themselves. The work of the ICDP allows care givers in developing and developed contexts alike to participate in reflective, empathic, caring interaction directed toward a very concrete expression of vulnerability (a child). To fully separate a liberal justice argument for responsibility from an approach based on caring and relationality, the question of 'motivation' to action remains an important one. The introduction of immersions (placing development workers within host families for a short period of time) represents a 'shallow' introduction to empathic understanding. The work of the ICDP, instead, is presented as a 'deep' application of empathic processes within both developed and developing communities.

In so far as the MDGs or any post-2015 variant are found to reflect a continuation of the neoliberal logic that suggests that there is 'an immanent free market essence to all societies' (Harrison, 2005, p 1307); in so far as the stated goals are depoliticised or reflect a compartmentalisation of 'targets' that fail to reflect the interconnected nature and structural reality of social inequalities of wealth, power and status; and in so far as such goals are supported by a theoretical framework of justice based on individual freedom, capabilities or rights, care theorists will continue to provide insight into the limits of such goals. In *The Cruel Choice*, development scholar Denis Goulet attempted to articulate an ethic of international development that took 'vulnerability' as its key focus. Unlike 'poverty' (the focus of much development intervention), vulnerability in societies was understood to reflect a lack of 'adequate defences against the social forces which propel them into the processes of change' (Goulet, 1971 [1985], p 38). It is not a lack or a want, but rather 'defenselessness, insecurity, and exposure to risks, shocks and stress' (Chambers, 1981, p 1). Within their own field, Goulet and Chambers were ahead of their time in making this important argument. And while in the interim a vast literature on care ethics in relation to human security has emerged, responsibility to concrete, embodied and intersubjective experiences of vulnerability in development contexts has not taken on the prominence that it should. While care ethics have contributed to our understanding of responsibility and attentiveness to caring needs, it is the co-responsibility and intersubjectivity within these relationships that a clearer focus on human empathy could provide. If the past 20 years of international development could be said to have reflected a focus on human development, then an ethics of care informed by a stronger appreciation for empathy could point us in the direction of a development of human *relationships,* thus strengthening the web of care within *and* across national boundaries.

Notes

[1] While throughout this piece I use the terms (international) development, development and human development, it is this last one that captures best the ethical discussion I am engaging in. In so far as the MGDs are based on a broadly conceived theory of justice (in the HCA), both can be seen to fall under the broader umbrella of the Human Development Approach. For Sen, human development requires 'advancing the richness of human life, rather than the richness of the economy in which human beings live' (see Shaikh, 2007, p 4). In so far as an ethic of care focuses on *relationships* of care, I suggest that it is consistent with this broader conception of human development while still an ideal critical corrective to the individual-oriented HCA.

[2] Mahbub ul Haq is founder of the UN Development Programme's *Human Development* reports.

[3]   This term is chosen specifically to draw a link with the *Buen Vivir or suma qamaña* movement in Bolivia, described by Arturo Escobar (Escobar, 1995 [2012]). Not simply an alternate vision of 'the good life' (in its more traditional, liberal sense), the pluriverse described by Escobar contains indigenous (read: local) understanding of a 'living well' that is at times non-liberal and non-capitalist; that incorporates ideas ('rights of nature', for example) that are outside of the standard 'civilisational' model of modernisation and development.

[4]   See note 1 above.

[5]   Pedwell herself, however, focuses mainly on 'affective' responses and at times refers to empathy (inconsistently with how I have attempted to explain it) as an 'emotion'.

[6]   This, however, consisted *also* with an HCA position, such as Nussbaum's, which argues that *all* nations, countries, communities are 'developing' communities, 'in that they contain problems of human development and struggles for a fully adequate quality of life and for minimal justice' (Nussbaum, 2011, p 16).

[7]   In psychoanalytic texts, double representation refers to the condition in which an empathic observer *feels* the affective or emotional state of another (single representation or sympathy) but then also recognises that feeling as coming from outside herself (see Agosta, 1984).

Section Two
Care ethics in practice

NINE

Exploring possibilities in telecare for ageing societies

Ingunn Moser and Hilde Thygesen

Introduction

A new focus on technology in health and care services is part of an international trend. The demographic changes implied by ageing populations, the growing chronicity of illness, together with rising expectations, lack of qualified labour and rising costs of public welfare are expected to pose challenges to public welfare systems. Policy responses to this impending 'care crisis' promote technology or 'telecare' as a solution that may at the same time reduce care needs and public expenditure *and* improve the quality of life of older people, by allowing them to receive the necessary support at home and to maintain their independence for as long as possible.

Critical engagements with these discourses note that there seems to be an underlying assumption that technology (for example GPS tracking technology, automatic alarms, detectors and medical monitoring devices) can replace the need for care and human relations and networks, and that this is seen to be desirable (Chaper One in this volume; see also Roberts and Mort, 2009; Mort et al, 2013). This policy is built on the assumption that people prefer to grow old in own their homes rather than living and being taken care of in institutions, and that technology will enable them to do so. These expectations of a 'technological fix' relate also to groups not previously considered as candidates for independent living, such as people with dementia.

From a care ethics perspective, the discourses of active ageing and independence and of a technological fix that replaces care needs and substitutes embodied , face-to-face, direct care with electronically mediated care at a distance seem to miss the point of care altogether. They contribute to the on-going individualisation of care (Chapter One in this volume) and also turn care issues into issues of individual risk management and security (Lopez, 2010). A central notion of care ethics, however, is the notion of the relational interdependence of people as caring subjects (Barnes, 2012a). According to Tronto (1993), people exist in and through caring relations with others. Care is constitutive of individual human being as well as of social and public life. People are relational entities, and so are their identities and subjective capacities. What characterises people is interdependence, rather than independence or dependence. Terms like relative or relational autonomy (MacKenzie and Stoljar, 2000) have been proposed to replace individualist notions of subjectivity, and autonomy and independence are analysed as relational achievements (Moser, 2006; 2011). On this basis, care ethics has delivered a powerful challenge to and critique of medical (principle) ethics and its ideal of individual, autonomous subjectivity (Verkerk, 1999). As Pols (2014) notes, it is hard to overestimate this achievement.

One could address the promotion of telecare development and its ideals in a similar way. Telecare discourse treats care first and foremost as expenditure, and care needs as a risk or even a threat to welfare budgets and future welfare systems. Much if not most telecare development is oriented towards reducing needs and the costs of care by teaching people to care and take responsibility for themselves, to manage their own risk profile and prevent their condition from deteriorating. On this basis, one could analyse policy and discourse, its philosophical and ideological frame, and reclaim the language and practice of care from telecare.

Policy and public discourse are important arenas when considering the shaping of future welfare provision, including the role of telecare. Even so, they are not the only relevant arenas. Policy and discourse do not tell the whole truth about telecare. In order to know what telecare is becoming, one has to take into account the everyday practices of caring relationships in people's lives. Care is a relational, situated and embodied achievement in which people explore the right thing to do for themselves and their relationships (Williams, 2004a). Accordingly, what makes good care varies. It is not a given, but becomes translated and negotiated in the concrete settings, arrangements and collectives that constitute care practice (Mol, Moser and Pols, 2010; Thygesen and Moser, 2010; Willems and Pols, 2010). Ethics of care practice therefore need to start from within care practice.

This chapter begins from these central notions of care ethics and by appreciating that questions about what constitutes good care, including telecare, cannot be tackled theoretically and in isolation from the actual context of care. Attempting to explore and shed light upon the phenomenon of telecare, and how it shapes and transforms care practice as well as values and ideals in care, requires that one undertakes empirical research into the practice and the aims and reflections of the actors involved, including patients, family care givers and healthcare practitioners (Pols, 2012). On this basis, then, empirically grounded ethics of care practice may articulate what really happens as well as what is striven for and achieved in actual practice. This may also be compared with practices and ideals in other care contexts, or in arenas such as policy or technological innovation. It may also provide material for reflection and debate and argument and reasoning about the value and quality of current care practices, and provide suggestions and recommendations (Willems and Pols, 2010).

This type of empirical ethics of care practice does not shun normativity, but places it at centre stage. Indeed, the question of the value and quality of a practice, of what to do and what is the good and right thing to do at any one time, is at the very heart of a care collective, and is very much what binds and holds a care collective together. This type of empirical ethics thus treats care practice as inherently normative and as a form of ethics-in-practice, and sees empirical ethics as taking part in the same discourse and on the same level, in the middle of practice (Thygesen, 2009).

Accordingly, this chapter illustrates, analyses and describes how telecare, exemplified by use of GPS-based tracking technology in care for people with dementia, establishes a form of care at a distance, and what this implies for different actors in the care collective. It traces what they strive for, how they weigh and balance, different values and ideals, what is achieved and how, and what conditions are essential for this achievement. It asks how telecare affects and possibly transforms care practice, care values and ideals, and divisions of labour and the distribution and assignment of responsibility. Finally, it explores the challenges, limitations and limits involved. The arguments are based upon empirical data drawn from an EU-funded research project on ethical frameworks for telecare for elderly people living at home).[1] The research is based on analyses of policy documents, debates in citizens' panels and ethnographical fieldwork and interviews about how these new caring solutions work in practice within formal healthcare services and in family care. For pedagogical reasons, we rely on excerpts from interviews and ethnographic field notes related to one single case. These excerpts, however, demonstrate and illustrate the more general lessons from EFORTT-project research (Roberts and Mort, 2009; Lopez, 2010; Mort et al, 2013).

Experimenting with telecare arrangements: affording valued positions, reciprocity and symmetry

Dementia is often described as the condition that exemplifies how illness strikes not only individual persons and patients, but whole families or care collectives. The following stories illustrate this. They are from an interview with a family carer who is talking about her husband's condition and their experiences when using a GPS-based tracking technology.

> "My husband was diagnosed with dementia five years ago. He has always gone for long walks, even after he became ill. The problems increased after a while. There were incidents when he got lost, and once he almost froze to death. Later, he turned the day around and started taking walks outside in the middle of the night. For a while I was out looking for him almost every night. It was a nightmare for both of us. I still had to get up for work every day! I dragged out my mattress, placed it in front of the entrance door and went to bed there in order to be able to prevent him from going out – only to find out that he had used the garden entrance instead. That's when I bought myself this GPS. It was connected both to mine and our daughter's mobile phone, and made it possible to find out where he was at all times. I have to admit it was like getting a new life for us both. Once again I was able to start exercising and join the choir. And my husband started to go out dancing, which he hadn't done for many years."

The above excerpt shows a family struggling to handle life with dementia. It further shows family carers experimenting with various care arrangements, including telecare. They are exploring possibilities and solutions for themselves, their caring relationships and their everyday lives. They try this and they try that, constantly tinkering and seeking good and better arrangements (Mol, Moser and Pols, 2010; Thygesen and Moser, 2010). We will analyse what this good or 'right thing' is for each of the participants in the care relationship and care collective at stake.

Per Hansen (to safeguard anonymity, we have used a fictitious name) had always been an 'outdoors' man with an active life-style, and was still in a good physical shape. When he fell ill with dementia it was out of the question for his wife and family to refuse him his freedom to move about as he was used to. During the early phase of the illness he had problems with orientation, which created challenges related to his safety, and daily (and nightly!) search and rescue actions for his family. The introduction of a GPS unit, however, made it possible for them to continue to care for Per at home for three more years, rather than handing him over to care in a sheltered (and locked) ward in a nursing home.

In a first reading and interpretation, then, what the GPS unit did was to make it possible for Per Hansen to continue to claim and exercise his individual freedom and, as part of this, his self-determination, independence and capacity to take care of himself. But perhaps more important was the fact that the GPS unit allowed Per to continue leading the life he was used to and maintain activities that had been important in shaping his identity. It created continuity with his previous life. He could enjoy nature – a source of aesthetic value, and to many people also of spiritual value. He could also maintain social relationships and he took up an old hobby and passion: dancing.

These activities, made possible by the GPS unit, gave him access to positions and relations that were not dependency related but built on reciprocity and interdependence. By visiting an old female friend he could, for example, show compassion and care, not just receive it. Taking part in such activities allowed Per to maintain his identity and a subjective self not defined by and reduced to the dementia disease and dependency. As such, it contributed to an evening-out of power asymmetries, or at least to bringing in more symmetry to some situations and relations.

The GPS unit opened up and afforded new positions and identities for Per Hansen's wife and family as well. It gave his wife and daughter the assurance of safety that they needed in order to maintain their work and financial responsibilities in addition to their caring responsibilities. Before the GPS unit came into their lives, Per's wife spent hours both day and night looking for him. With the GPS technology, Per's movements could be followed from a distance, and she could go out to fetch him home if it became too late, if he got exhausted or if he couldn't find his way home. She was no longer constantly worn out, but could start exercising and attending choir practice again. She was no longer reduced to and fixed in a position as carer. In this way, the GPS unit 'unfixed' the dyadic positions of carer and care recipient in their relationship. So, in this case, bringing a new element into the care collective opened up valued positions and enabled some more symmetry and reciprocal interdependence for all involved.

Telecare comes with new demands and responsibilities

We have seen above the positive effect of telecare in affording a whole new life to a family care collective. But telecare also comes with new demands and responsibilities that may be challenging to take on.

> "I had regular routines for charging the GPS. I was terrified to forget, so I charged it every evening, even though it wasn't necessary. Afterwards, before going to bed, I attached it to the belt on his trousers, since he always put those on when he got up. In that way I knew he wouldn't lose it.
>
> "[...] By using technical solutions, we transfer an additional responsibility. My responsibility was to ensure that the GPS unit was charged. If not, and it got discharged when he used it, it was my fault if something happened. It was also up to me to find a way to make sure he took it with him."

Per's wife is a healthcare professional, and sees the consequences and challenges implied by new technologies from the viewpoint of both the healthcare worker and the family carer. In this quote, she reflects on her responsibility as a family carer and the new tasks and solutions she has to carry out. As she says, the new caring solutions come with certain requirements: someone has to ensure that the unit is charged, that it is switched on, that it doesn't get switched off if someone touches it, that it is not so cold that the batteries discharge while Per is outside, that the device is brought back and isn't left on a tree stump during a break or removed from Per's backpack. If these conditions are not present, the current arrangement will not work and the technology will not provide protection or security.

Per Hansen's wife experimented with and tried out several creative solutions to ensure that things would work. She made routines for charging the GPS unit. After an incident where Per took the GPS unit out of his backpack or jacket pocket, she first tried putting the unit in a leather pouch attached to his keyring. Finally, her solution was to attach it to the belt of his trousers. In addition, she found a means of protecting the power button so as to prevent Per from switching the unit off by accident.

When the person with a particular need for care and for new care arrangements and solutions is living at home, he or she is the family's responsibility. This is experienced as a demanding responsibility, one that does not surface in the telecare debates. Telecare also adds further demands and responsibilities, and not all families and relatives have the means to handle them. Many elderly relatives have little experience with new technology. When it comes to GPS, numerous solutions are available on the commercial market and it is no easy task for family carers to choose the best solution, operator or supplier unassisted.

Telecare creates new work and requires new skills and routines

When Per moved to the local nursing home after some years, it was uncertain whether he would be allowed to keep the GPS. The staff had no experience in this area and contacted the county governor for clarification. Fortunately, the county governor approved Per Hansen's use of the GPS relatively quickly. Today Per still goes for long walks, generally every day, and now the staff at the nursing home monitor his location.

> "Now I log in [to the PC] and track him around lunchtime to see where he is located and if he is on his way back. If I see there is a movement in the right direction, I wait for a while to see if he shows up by himself. A couple of times we have had to go out and get him. A while ago, for example, I discovered that he was in the same place when I checked again about half an hour later. Then I took my car and went to find him. Apparently he was quite exhausted, and had taken a break. But evidently he felt comfortable getting a ride back here."

This quote is from an interview with the unit manager at the nursing home where Per Hansen is living. She is describing how they use and integrate the GPS unit, what the implications are and how the new tasks, responsibilities, skills and routines are handled. In this particular excerpt she describes how the staff log on to a computer or mobile phone to find out where Per is, and the discretionary judgements involved in deciding what to do. They check his position, and later on check which direction he is moving in. When they see his position on the screen they make several professional evaluations. Where is he, how far has he gone, how long has he been out, is he on his way back, what is his condition and is it necessary to go and get him? These are some of the questions the staff need to consider on the basis of the information on the computer screen. This is not a new task, but one that is performed in a different way and that requires new and different skills because the staff have to read and interpret Per's condition in an electronically mediated way. The screen is a new instrument through which they have to learn to see and read their resident and patient's condition – and the resident is not directly present, for instance to ask him questions.

In addition, those responsible for Per Hansen's care make several other professional and discretionary evaluations on a daily basis. For example, they have to evaluate whether the weather is too cold for him to go out, despite having the GPS. And they have to evaluate traffic safety.

But there are also entirely new tasks: the GPS unit has to be charged, it must be put in the backpack or attached to his belt, someone has to check on his position and condition, and sometimes one of the staff has to drive out to bring Per Hansen home. There are also new administrative routines related to new technologies because they are subject to specific guidelines related to privacy regulations, for instance.

In the nursing home, clear definitions of both task performance and responsibility are required for the GPS unit. This is stipulated in more or less formal procedures. At Per's nursing home the night nurse is responsible for charging the GPS unit each night. A 'charging list' has been posted on the wall in the guardroom and has to be signed each time. The primary daytime contact is responsible for ensuring that the GPS is switched on and that Per Hansen has it with him when he goes for a walk. The nursing home staff put the GPS unit in with his water bottle in the pouch that he carries around his waist and always takes with him. Per's primary contact is also responsible for checking his position, monitoring him and evaluating his condition, and keeping track of him, either through the computer or by mobile phone, while he is out walking.

Weighing and balancing different values and ideals in care

> "But I am terrified that it [the GPS] doesn't work. It gets dark in two hours. And the message is sent. But I don't know why his unit doesn't answer. The batteries could be discharged. Or perhaps he has accidentally switched it off. Or there could be something wrong with the subscription."

Again, Per Hansen's wife is reflecting. She is speaking about the 'technological risks' involved in telecare, risks that cannot be separated from human or organisational risks. This is about delegating, and handing over the task and responsibility for direct clinical observation and monitoring of a patient's condition to machines or technical instruments. Large segments of specialised healthcare now delegate and rely on machines for monitoring certain functions or parameters. In this sense, telecare builds on and extends practices that are familiar. Telecare has something else in common with specialised healthcare, and this is that machines and instruments often see and monitor conditions that are not so easily or directly accessible to traditional clinical observation. Their observations may penetrate more deeply into the person and body's condition, and more broadly into the person's situation and context. As such, the use of technical instruments and machines in (health)care makes new things possible. Still, the distance at which telecare operates is new and different in its reach. In addition, telecare, including the use of GPS in dementia care, is new and is reliant on experimentation and 'learning in action'. Our experience with it so far is limited.

Even so, what is important to Per Hansen's wife is that Per can remain active and go for walks in the forest, maintain a way of life that defines a crucial part of his identity and experience continuity with his previous life. This is more important than security in its traditional meaning in care, or that she herself feels that Per's safety is maintained. What the GPS technology affords in this situation is a new form of security for an activity and practice that until now has not been a component of, or even conceivable within, care. There are no resources at the nursing home to follow residents outdoors for hours on end. Locking physically strong residents into closed units creates frustration and sometimes anger and despair in patients who can neither defuse their energy nor fulfil their intentions when incarcerated. The last thing that Per's wife wants is for her husband to be stuck in a closed unit.

But also for her own sake, it is important to have independence and the possibility to maintain a life beyond disease and care-taking responsibility. "The GPS made it possible for me to go to work," she says. She "got a new life", or got her life back, and was no longer totally bound by her care-taking responsibilities, since she didn't have to be physically present all the time. In that way, the GPS technology and the care it provided represented care for both her and Per, to the family as well as to the person who was defined as being in need of care.

What, then, about the staff at the nursing home? As already stated, locking residents up in closed units creates tensions and conflict between residents, and between residents and staff. This is part of the reality that needs to be dealt with in such a unit and that requires energy and resources – relational, emotional and mental. The dilemma is that on the one hand there are neither the time nor the resources to fulfil residents' individual needs – for instance for outdoor physical activity – but that if the residents are just allowed to go out, the staff may be held responsible for neglect of care. On the other hand, carers are not happy with the situation of frustrated and despairing residents who cannot fulfil their needs. Here too there is an element of neglect, but the issue of safety and security has traditionally weighed more heavily than individual fulfilment. Telecare, however, promises to take care of safety and security and thereby make room for other values, such as enjoying valued positions and relations: nature, friendship, self-determination. The priorities and values of safety, security and individual fulfilment are no longer in conflict – or at least, the options are no longer so clear cut. With the use of the GPS unit, Per Hansen's individual needs and his security are both taken care of. Accordingly, Per can use his physical energy in a more constructive way than by simply walking restlessly back and forth along closed corridors, and frustration can be replaced by fulfilment.

The introduction of the GPS unit forced a rethinking of patient safety and security and patient protection. The staff consulted the county governor for clearance and advice. For the county governor, the critical question was whether the new telecare arrangements implied improper monitoring. For the healthcare staff, however, the critical issue was whether the new arrangements could be trusted. Watching residents is a critical part of their job, and delegating this task and responsibility to a technical device such as the GPS unit seemed to be a real-time experiment. When the patient leaves the enclosed environment of the institution, care provision must now operate under new, unfamiliar and uncertain conditions. There is the difficulty of monitoring and limiting possible risks; and technological monitoring alone does not secure anything. Monitoring has to be accompanied and followed up by interpretation, discretionary judgement and action – and preparedness for action in terms of resources, procedures and routines. At the time of our interviews, the staff at the nursing home were busy developing and testing such procedures, routines and preparedness.

Until recently, people with dementia were not considered to have the same needs or to be capable of living active, social, self-determined and independent lives. However, this is changing. People with dementia are now expected to have a voice in matters concerning their own care and to be entitled to individual and personalised care. It is in this situation that telecare enters the arena. The values and ideals as such are not new or specific to telecare, and do not depend on the introduction of technology in and of itself. But telecare arrangements and solutions highlight and also recursively add to and strengthen the current discourses that contribute to individualised care – in more than one sense.

Conclusion: is telecare replacing or relying on care and networks?

This chapter has described how telecare opens up valued positions and relations, but also involves new tasks, skills, responsibilities, procedures and routines, preparedness and resources, weighing and balancing of benefits and priorities, creative solutions and negotiations, so as to make things work out and work together. This applies to family care as well as to institutional and professional care provision. In our final quote we return to Per Hansen's wife.

> "When I ordered the GPS, there were several hitches. The supplier programmed it ready for use. All I had to do was to arrange the telephone subscriptions, one for him and one for me. But then the phone operator did something with the subscription and suddenly it didn't work.
>
> "I had a regular mobile phone subscription and started two new ones when we bought the GPS. That meant that three mobile phone numbers appeared when people searched for my number in the internet phone register. Naturally, they didn't know which numbers were valid. A friend of mine sent a text message to the GPS. I called the telephone operator and told them that this number should be hidden. However, they closed the number on his GPS by mistake and this caused his GPS to malfunction. The supplier discovered this by accident. All we knew was that the GPS wasn't working as it should. Finally, the supplier called the telephone operator and sorted things out."

This story emphasises once again that if telecare solutions are to work, someone has to facilitate, coordinate and take responsibility. It also tells us that new participants come into the picture – in this case, equipment suppliers and telephone operators. As this shows, they become involved in and are a part of the care collective. They are involved in those facilitations, practices and processes that at any given time support Per Hansen as a resident and patient, and help to create the conditions for the capacities, qualifications, positions and possibilities that he is given.

In the political rhetoric surrounding telecare, the argument that technology represents a new solution, especially for those with no family or social network, is often used. Technology is supposed to replace a network or a collective that can take care of you. Technology is supposed to make it possible for those standing alone to continue to care for themselves. Indeed, taking care of oneself emerges as the most prominent value and ideal in care, according to telecare.

This rhetoric is in sharp contrast to the telecare practices that our research discovered. Our studies show that technologies don't work in a vacuum or by themselves. On the contrary, they require a collective of diverse participants, a coordination and distribution of tasks and responsibilities, development and formalisation of procedures, routines and skills, and the availability and commitment of resources to provide capacity for action. Either the technology has to be incorporated into an existing care collective, as in Per's case, or a new one has to be mobilised, defined and joined up. Within this care collective, participants must be qualified and made responsible. For example, somebody must be assigned the task of ordering a telephone subscription, be a contact for suppliers and operators, arrange the listing in the telephone catalogue and sort things out if the technology is not providing the information about the person's whereabouts because the subscription has been blocked by mistake. As we have seen previously, somebody has to recharge the batteries, follow up and learn to observe and interpret information in new ways. And somebody has to take on the task of looking for or fetching the patient when he doesn't find his way home.

To sum up: telecare does not replace people with technology and monitoring. Care is not put aside or diminished. Care can be mediated and activated from a distance. And technologies may also challenge and change relations of power, and allow for new dynamics and new, valued positions and identities. Telecare involves new possibilities, but it also has limitations. Technologies do not work by themselves and accomplish everything by themselves. There are many tasks and functions that cannot be delegated to technologies alone. As we have shown, somebody has to perform a variety of tasks that create the conditions for the technologies to work. Not everyone can take on these tasks or carry these responsibilities, and not everyone has someone who can take on these tasks and responsibilities for them.

Acknowledgements

We would like to thank users, family members and staff in dementia care who willingly shared their experiences in the EFORTT-project. The research in this project, on which this chapter is based, was made possible through funds from the EU's Seventh Framework Programme. We are also very grateful to our international partners and colleagues in the project.

Note

[1] The project Ethical Frameworks for Telecare Technologies for Older People at Home involved researchers from Spain, the Netherlands, Great Britain and Norway and was financed through the EU's Seventh Framework Programme. The project lasted from 2008 to 2011. See www.lancs.ac.uk/efortt.

TEN

Paradoxical constructions in Danish elder care

Anne Liveng

Introduction

Transformations are taking place in Danish elder care that have consequences for both older citizens and care workers. These transformations are connected to economic concerns and to scientifically and ideologically based changes in how older people are perceived, and they are shaping the support offered to older people by the welfare state. This chapter focuses on the consequences of different philosophical conceptualisations of human beings; specifically, on the ways in which older people are viewed and how this influences ideas both about the care they may need and about how professionals should behave towards old people in need of support. This interest reflects a general concern about how neoliberalism, with its conception of human beings as rational, independent, free-choosing customers, changes the role of the state and, through 'technologies of the self', moves caring responsibilities away from the community and onto the individual. It is argued that the discourse of active ageing changes the concept and practice of care when it is implemented as policy for elder care. Neoliberal conceptualisations of what it is to be human question fundamental principles of the Nordic welfare state model, which has been characterised by a mutual responsibility for all citizens based on universal welfare principles and a high degree of economic redistribution. Drawing on empirical material from a study of activity centres for older citizens, the chapter shows how macro-level policies and organisational framing pervade norms, values and practice on a micro level.

Older people who are too frail, ill or lonely to be on their own at home during the day time can attend activity centres either voluntarily or by municipal referral. The empirical material for this chapter is drawn from an evaluation of a learning project for care workers in activity centres and consists of interviews with care workers, observations of daily situations in the centres, and notes of the researcher's own thoughts and emotions in connection to the observations. The care workers in this study were critical of neoliberal notions of human beings, and expressed feelings of infringement when they felt their experience based knowledge from at work were being ignored. And, as the care workers explain and the observations illustrate, the lives of the older people in question are not always in harmony with the idea of the resourceful, active and independent elder that is presented in the new image. To understand this, it is necessary to turn to theories encompassing the fundamental concept of human interdependence and need for care, which is life long but which becomes obvious especially in older age.

Care and recognition

Care ethics and Axel Honneth's theory of recognition are predicated on human interconnectedness. They both aim to establish a theoretical framework that is able to link micro and macro levels, and they both provide a foundation for critique of the neoliberal ideologies that are currently permeating welfare states (Lloyd, 2012). Whereas care ethics connects care and justice, Honneth links recognition and justice (Honneth, 2004; Barnes, 2012a). These two theoretical orientations provide a basis for thorough analyses and critique of the above-mentioned transformation processes.

Honneth's theory of recognition has its roots in the German Frankfurt School. From a starting point anchored in anthropology and philosophy, Honneth (2007) defines recognition as a basic human need that is crucial for human individuation. Social acknowledgement takes place in an interpersonal space – as human beings we are able to keep up a positive relationship to ourselves only through the confirming and approving reactions of other subjects. The ability to sense, interpret and realise one's needs and desires as a fully individuated person depends crucially on the development of self-confidence, self-respect and self-esteem. The three modes of relating practically to oneself are acquired and maintained inter-subjectively when one is granted recognition by someone whom one also recognises, in three spheres of recognition.

1. The sphere of love: the mutual emotional contact in intimate social relations such as love relationships, family or friendship, imparted through love and care provides the human being with ontological safety and self-confidence. This recognition stands out as

a precondition for the ability to enter inter-subjective relationships at all.

2. The sphere of rights: the legal acceptance as a moral and 'sane' member of a society through respect and universal rights provides the individual with self-respect.

3. The sphere of solidarity: the social valuation of individual abilities, involvement and participation in a community through solidarity results in self-esteem.

Lack of recognition leads on the subjective level to experiences of infringement; on the societal level to the disintegration of society. On the basis of 'people's experiences of infringement, Honneth argues, it is possible to form a critique of developments in society and formulate visions of 'the good life'.

Writers in the tradition of care ethics take the relation of care itself as a point of departure for their political critique of the neoliberal conception of the human being. A need for care is seen as inherent in the human condition, which means that ideas about citizenship, equity and social justice are closely linked to equal access to and possibilities for receiving care, on the one hand, and motivation for and meaningfulness in caring for fellow human beings, on the other (Lloyd, 2012). The gender perspective is an integrated dimension of the critique, as the care deficit on both a national and a global level has unequal consequences for women and men (see Tronto, Chapter Two in this volume).

Turning to the area of elder care, care and recognition seem to be two sides of the same coin. When Tronto defined care in *Moral Boundaries* (1993), she described four phases, in which the recognition of the care-needing subject is central. 'Caring about' implies recognition of a need for care. Often, Tronto suggests, it will involve assuming the position of the person or group in question in order to recognise the need. In the article 'Invisibility', Honneth (2001) explains the difference between cognitive awareness of another person and recognition. 'Caring about' has strong similarities with this description of recognition, as it implies a positive attitude towards and affirmation of the other person. 'Taking care of' involves taking responsibility for and responding to the need. Most often this will require some sort of action that is also present in 'care-giving', as it involves the direct meeting of the needs and contact between the care giver and the recipient of care. Finally, 'care-receiving' is the element in the process that provides the only way to know that caring needs have been met. The quality of the four phases of care is dependent on the care giver's ability to recognise and be empathic towards the other person and her needs, and claims that caring will not be fulfilled until the care giver is positively confirmed by the care receiver of her needs being met. This process involves elements of the recognition provided in Honneth's sphere of love, and elements of recognition in the sphere of solidarity as the care receiver's ability to evaluate and appreciate the act of caring is acknowledged. In addition, it involves practical acts; so that while recognition is an integrated element in the processes of caring, caring also requires *more* than a recognising attitude.

Changing views on older people

In recent decades elder care in Denmark has been organised on the basis of principles and methods deriving from New Public Management (NPM) (Dahl, 2011). The aim has been to rationalise and increase the effectiveness of care work and thereby reduce the cost of welfare services. With a rapidly growing number of older people in Denmark, it is argued that rationalisation is necessary in order to prevent frail elders from becoming an increasing economic burden (Kamp and Hvid, 2012). The focus has been on the care providers: on the role and responsibilities of local authorities and, in terms of the purchaser–provider model, on the role and responsibilities of care workers and management.

During the past decade a political shift in focus from care providers to the receivers of care has taken place. Major local authorities develop programmes for older people under slogans such as 'Active all your life'. In policy documents the differences between groups of older people are presented, together with the possibilities for older people to continue making their own choices in order to live a meaningful and healthy life. Policies for including and activating older citizens so as to take care of their life and health are developed; for example, as strategies for rehabilitation in home-based care for older people. Older people are spoken of as having resources that the professionals have to draw on. Dahl (2011, p 148) speaks of a 'radicalization' of the ideal of self-determination in public documents in the 2000s, which goes hand in hand with a division of older people into two groups, the self-determined and the frail (Barnes, 2012a).

A background for this division can be found in two separate developments in gerontology: the distinction between 'third age' and 'fourth age' and the distinction between 'successful' and 'normal' ageing.

The concepts of third and fourth age were formulated by Laslett (1989) as a way of distinguishing between older people who have left work due to retirement but are self-reliant and strong in resources, and those who need support from others to manage their everyday life. In Western countries the life phase after retirement is longer than ever before in history, and Laslett's distinction functions as a tool to enhance the understanding of differences between groups of people belonging to this life phase.

The debate in gerontology on successful ageing was initiated by Rowe and Kahn (1997). In their terminology, 'successful ageing' represents an ideal of ageing not necessarily as a process influenced by decay and loss, but as a stage of life with maintenance of high cognitive and physical functional ability. This ability is to be reached through the individual's own mastering of health by engagement in physical and social activity. 'Normal ageing', in contrast, describes the common idea of ageing – and very often also the reality, at least for the oldest old – as a period of life when one is becoming more fragile, affected by illnesses and dependent on the support of others. Critical gerontologists have argued that the ideal of successful ageing is historically and culturally constructed (Katz, 2000) and that the possibility for living a 'successful old life' is unequally distributed according to class, gender and ethnicity (Holstein and Minkler, 2003; see Ward, L., Chapter Four in this volume).

From gerontology to the elder care sector

In the Danish elder care sector the image of the third age and the ideas expressed in the theory of successful ageing have entered into policy and practice. Supported by numerous quantitative investigations showing the connection between physical activity, functional ability and health, 'successful ageing' has turned into the discourse of 'active ageing'. As Dahl (2011) argues in her article 'Who Can Be Against Quality?' central words used in the NPM discourse are empty signifiers that it is impossible to debate as their denotation is only positive. Thus the term 'active' has no negative connotations; it is a positive but empty signifier, as the word itself tells us nothing about how you are supposed to be active.

The shift from considering older people who come into contact with municipal elder care services as people in need of care because of frailty or illness, to viewing them as persons who can be motivated and are able to improve both their health and level of activity, has resulted in new municipal strategies. In policy documents aimed at older citizens, the quality of life and independence connected with an active (and thereby healthy life) are emphasised. In Denmark the Municipality of

Fredericia has been in the forefront of this movement. On the municipal website the leaflet 'Active all Life' can be found. The leaflet presents the values of Fredericia municipality and the initiatives organised in relation to older people. The municipality wants 'to break with the traditional thinking, [...] that to be old is in itself a sign of lacking resources and being dependent on support' (author's translation). 'Quality of life', making one's own decisions, taking responsibility and help to self-help are key words. 'It doesn't make sense to define people on the basis of their age', the leaflet states. Therefore the municipality has not developed a specific elders policy, 'but a policy for the services offered to all citizens who have a reduced functional ability'. The first page ends by concluding that 'older people, like everybody else, are covered by the vision for Fredericia of citizens taking responsibility'.It is easy to see this text as expressing respect for the individual human being, who, rather than being regarded as a more or less passive 'client' in the dominant discourse is now put in the centre of the welfare services as a responsible and autonomous person. But it contains both paradoxes and statements that are so self-evident that they seem odd. Of course age *in itself* is not tantamount to lacking resources or losing functional ability. But age *is* connected to both illnesses and wearing out of the body that can lead to reduced abilities (Lloyd, 2012). It seems that the municipality is both denying and accepting this at one and the same time. Why offer older people the same services as other citizens with 'reduced functional abilities' if there is no acceptance of the connection between old age and frailty? Or, to put it differently, if there is no acceptance of 'normal ageing' as the common condition of ageing? The emphasis on the autonomy and self-responsibility of older people is also peculiar. Is it not self-evident that adults prefer to manage their own lives and to be independent of public support for as long as possible? Why this strong demand for something that most citizens, as the leaflet itself states, already practise?

Higgs et al (2009) argue from a governmentality perspective that the stress on self-responsibility can be understood as an example of how health-related 'technologies of the self' enter into later life. These technologies aim to enhance the self-government of older individuals because of concerns about the economic impact of increasing numbers of older people. The longer that the fluid line between third and fourth age can be extended, the less expensive municipal elder care will be. If 'normal ageing' can be turned into 'successful ageing' by making citizens take responsibility for living a physically and socially active life, it may be possible to reduce public expense.

Seen from the perspective of care ethics, this movement challenges the collective responsibility for taking care of those who cannot care for themselves that has been characteristic of Nordic welfare states. The insistent focus on one's own responsibility suggests that people have to be motivated to take responsibility. In the light of the theory of recognition, this questioning represents potential limitations in the sphere of solidarity, because a precondition of this sphere is that each should contribute with their own resources and abilities and be recognised for their contribution. The emphasis on self-responsibilisation thus potentially plants a seed of mistrust towards those who are in need of public support. It may increase feelings of guilt among citizens who are not able to manage on their own and become dependent on public support. Fourth-age older people are in this group.

A 'paradigm shift' in day care centres

In 2007, like many other Danish councils, Copenhagen City Council adopted a new ageing policy. Following this policy, health and care authorities developed the project 'From day-care facilities to activity facilities', aimed at transforming day care centres in accordance with the ideas of active ageing. The project was labelled a paradigm shift in its approach to working with older people attending the centres and it involved competence development courses for all care workers. These courses were evaluated on the basis of observations and group interviews and the following examples stem from this empirical material (Liveng and Andersen, 2011). Methodologically, the research applied a reflective ethnographic approach (Davies, 1999), where both what happened in the 'outer world' and the feelings and reflections of the researchers were hermeneutically analysed.

Day care centres are often situated in municipal nursing homes, where they share kitchen facilities and dining halls. Most of the professionals, as well as service users, are women. At present, centres are struggling with declining occupancy. In order to make day care centres more attractive, their name was changed to 'activity centres', with variation in the specific activities offered in each. Each centre was expected to send older people to the other centres on the basis of the interests expressed by the older people themselves. The assessment rules were changed so that only citizens with severely reduced functional abilities were referred to centres through the council's assessment system. Other older people had to go to the centres on their own initiative and the centres became economically dependent on the number of citizens they could attract.

In order to meet new demands for evidence-based work, registration was introduced for those using the centres and it became a daily task for employees to enter information about the health and social conditions of older people into the municipal data system. Employees were offered competence development courses in order to learn about the ideas and practices of the scheme. Part of the curriculum was Antonovsky's salutogenic theory. This theory was developed in opposition to pathogenic theory and deals with the factors that keep people healthy, rather than those that make people ill. Employing the central term 'Sense of Coherence', it focuses on the single individual's experience of meaningfulness. A person's 'Sense of Coherence' is considered to be established in early adult life even though it is not unchangeable it is less dependent on the actual context or of relationships later in life.

Customers or members?

The activity paradigm created confusion among the health professionals about how to refer to older people attending the centres. On the courses, employees were taught to refer to them as 'members'. The argument for this choice of words was that now the least fragile people had to register by themselves as members in the specific activity centre they attended. But none of the employees spoke of the older people attending the centres as 'members' in the interviews. There were, however, striking shifts in discourse regarding the terms used for these older people, depending on the context and role in which they were seen. They were referred to as 'citizens' and 'users'; however, when talked about in relation to economic matters, they were 'customers':

> "I don't believe the other centres will send customers to us. It's something of a dilemma. Of course one would like to share the citizens, but we need customers. As it is now, you think mainly of yourself, that you have to get new customers, but if you imagine that it works so that it [the new activity programme] actually attracts more people, like that, then it will be obvious that you refer people to the others."

Different logics collide in the way employees see older people. Are they 'citizens', with all the connotations that this concept entails, such as people who are, in principle, equal to the employees, with the same human rights; or are they 'customers', people that the health professionals have to attract and make a living by? Citizens are people one would like to share, but customers are needed in the competition between centres. The commercialisation that the centres are forced into in order to survive financially apparently overturns the discourse of membership. The fact that about half of the older people are still referred to the centres by the municipality's assessment system because of vulnerability and reduced functional abilities seems to disappear in the new economic context. The quotation shows how the economic reality of the centres intrudes on the relationship between employees and older people. Likewise, it also changes the role of the professional person from that of a care worker to a kind of salesperson. But the very reason for having the centres is an unmet need for care among older citizens in the community, and the core task of the centre is to provide care, company and meaningfulness for those who are not able to establish this on their own. How can the professional recognise and meet the needs of these older citizens if they are seen as customers? From the perspective of care ethics, the discourse stands in the way of establishing a process of caring, as it does not provide an understanding of the dependency of the people in question.

At the same time the discourse contradicts the experiences of the professionals. While it is an economic reality for the centres that they have to attract 'customers', freely choosing customers is not what employees face in practice.

> "Now the elderly have to join the centre on their own initiative. The new elderly who are on the internet, they will find us. But we've always had difficulty filling up the day centres. Old people, they sit at home. They don't have the energy."

As in the leaflet from Fredericia municipality, paradoxical images are reflected in this quotation. The image of 'the new elders' who are searching the internet, looking for activities on offer, fits in well with the activity paradigm – and with the image of third-age older people. But another aspect of the reality of ageing is revealed: some of the older people are in fact unable to live up to the ideal of being active and self-choosing individuals. They are tired, and withdraw from social activities outside the house. Confusion about who is the target group of the centres appears: is it the resourceful, self-reliant citizens or is it those who need support in order to turn up? Centres are situated in old people's homes and partly integrated into the municipal assessment system, which indicates that the target group for the centres are fourth-age older people who are dependent on care-giving support. But, like the commercialisation of the centres, the activity paradigm potentially distorts the ability of the professionals to see and recognise the realities of the fourth age.

Is care needed?

Other employees speak with frustration about the city council's not knowing who the older people in question are. The humiliation felt by the professionals who feel that their knowledge is not recognised intertwines with worry for those whom they have to take care of.

> "They do not know how weak they are, how little most of them are able to do by themselves. Why didn't they ask us? We have not been heard."

Observations from the centres challenge the idea of 'the new active elders', too. They show the frailty of the older people attending and unfold the heavy emotional content present in the everyday situations. And they challenge the idea that meaningfulness can be found by a person independently of the context and life circumstances linked to old age:

> After lunch the old people sit down around the tables, some in their wheelchairs. The tables are still covered with paper, tape, yarn, etc for making Christmas decorations. Some of the older people continue their work; others just sit with their coffee cups in front of them, still others slowly begin to fall asleep. One member of the health professionals is at the tables; she shows some ladies a way of knitting pixies. Usually I enjoy making decorations, but now I almost experience nausea by looking at the pixies. I feel tired and think this will be a long afternoon. To do something I ask the lady sitting next to me if she doesn't want to make decorations. She looks at me in what I perceive a sarcastic way. 'No,' she says, 'I don't find it fun anymore. I've done so much, but now, what's the point? I'm the only one left. It's no fun anymore.' She turns away and I feel a kind of emptiness; what can you possibly answer to that? (Researcher's observation, December 2010)

This scene illustrates important aspects of the everyday situations among very old people in a day care centre. Even though 'activity' takes place, tiredness, hopelessness and withdrawal are also part of the reactions among the older people, and therefore what the professionals face in their daily work. In this context the notion of older people as active, independent individuals does not support care relations, as it does not contain an awareness of what is needed by the individual older person. Neither is the fourth phase of care – responsiveness – present, as the workers are not attentive to how the person is responding to the 'care' that is being given.

Care or documentation?

Employees, who have been working in the centres for several years declare that the personal contact with older people is the most important aspect of their work. They see older people as their 'guests' and have an awareness of their well-being as the core concern of their work.

> Employee: "That is what we feel is frustrating in connection to documentation, we have both to fill out questionnaires and to document, so we spend a lot of time away from our guests. And we do not have that time. I do not know what to document. How am I able to tell how they are, I haven't had time to talk to them, because I have been documenting? I think that is frustrating. And I think it is more important to talk to them than to get a whole lot written ..."

The logic of evidence-based work, which is the aim of documentation, collides with a relational understanding of care as something 'done' by talking and 'being together with' – what Tronto (2013) has described as 'caring with' or solidarity between carer and cared-for. The wish to spend time with older people suggests a different attitude than the objectification entailed by measuring through questionnaires. From the perspective of Tronto's four phases of care, 'being together with' can be seen as a prerequisite for 'caring about', as it is through daily interactions that needs for care become evident. Measuring the state of health of the older person through questionnaires entails an understanding of older people as people who are always in a position to be able to express their needs and state of health verbally or in writing. This is not automatically the case when it comes to individual older people.

Critical employees question the control involved in questionnaires and the 'surplus' knowledge deriving from health data registering systems. This knowledge has not been revealed directly to the health professionals by the older people themselves, they find it unethical to use it in their work. They argue that this knowledge can prevent them from meeting the older person openly and on equal terms. It can distort the relationship with the older person if, as employees, they have access to information that has been given that is not in the social context of the centre. To them, the standardised registration inhibits the care relation as a meeting between – in principle – equals.

From 'servicing' to activating

The employees all state that the activity concept will change their relationships with older people, independently of whether they see this change as positive or as destroying the care relation. In connection with the relationships, the focus is on the question of how much to 'offer services' rather than 'to activate' and 'to demand'. The employees present different attitudes to this question. Some find the concept destructive of the very essence of their work. In other cases it becomes clear how the activity discourse potentially functions as a shield against the fragility of older people. These employees talk about how they have been *'over responsible'* previously, and have done many things that the older people themselves could have done. In one interview, the interviewer notes an aggressive tone, which is also apparent in an ironical use of concepts of care: "*We have to keep the nursing thing out of it.*" In Danish the word 'nursing' describes care that is 'too much', in other words, care that resembles spoiling or waiting on someone.

The employees have learned the importance of 'putting up boundaries' and rejecting the expectations of older people. The way of working practised previously is abandoned, with reference to the professionals as having 'serviced' older people. Older people have almost behaved as spoiled children, who now have to be brought up to take responsibility for their own lives. The employees now demand self-responsibility from older people, and apparently some see this as a relief from a burden they previously bore themselves:

> "Before I would have taken the lady in the wheelchair instead of making her take the speaker's chair, I would have thought it's better for her to be driven than to walk by herself. When should we offer support and when are they able to do it by themselves? This approach has been changed during the courses.
>
> "[...] And that's what we need to work on, putting demands on them to take care of their own lives. It's you

who should decide, it's you who want to be here. It's not for my sake you come here. It is and must be for your own sake. And it seems to me that they have accepted these demands very well."

These statements illustrate how confrontation with the bodily and mental decay connected with the fourth age can raise anxiety (Twigg, 2006). The new ideologies and practices of work offer a theoretical and organisational support for establishing psychological limits between the care workers and older people. Thus the activity ideology moves 'the care giver burden' from employees onto older people. An understanding of the older people attending the centres as people who *are able as long as they want* represents a denial of the 'negative' but unavoidable sides of ageing. When employees identify with this understanding their role changes from that of care givers to that of motivators. Instead of recognising the needs of the older people, they mistrust the signs of dependency and refuse to provide care.

Conclusion

The analysis shows how the fusion of ideas deriving from gerontology and economic concerns changes the concept of care. The individualistic and rationalistic theories of human beings implied in the image of active elders deny the basic human interdependency that is especially evident in the fourth age. The construction of people in need of care as customers, with a free will and ability if they want, challenges care as a practice carried out in public institutions. The fusion of commercialisation and the activity ideology turns care workers into a paradoxical combination of salespersons, authoritarian child rearers, personal coaches and municipal controllers. The fusion can potentially lead to bad care practices, as it squeezes recognition of the individual person out of the interaction. As the interviews show, this is not the vision of the care workers, who also express experiences of infringement. The care workers themselves do not feel recognised in their work when they have to adapt to these constructions.

The application of care ethics might help practitioners in this situation to challenge the model that is being imposed. The situation calls for a re-evaluation of the concept of care; and for a conceptualisation of human beings as fundamentally interdependent. Such a process of 'renewal' could, as argued by Sevenhuijsen (2003), develop from theories of an ethic of care. Both care ethics and the theory of recognition offer alternatives to neoliberal thinking. By insisting on our mutual interdependency these theories take back responsibility to those who are in a position to take it, and offer care workers a central role in supporting the quality of life for people in the fourth age. The theory of recognition pays attention to the need for recognition among those who (carry out) care. In relation to practice, care ethics (through Tronto's elements of good care) may function as a guideline and provide points of awareness for care workers.

This chapter has dealt with elder care, but the ideology embedded in the described transformations potentially affects all citizens. Without an alternative understanding of the human condition, the basic purpose of a welfare state disappears.

ELEVEN

Contours of matriarchy in care for people living with AIDS

Anke Niehof

Every distinct account of care brings with it a particular focus, and it is desirable to have many such accounts. (Tronto, 2013, p 20)

Introduction

The conventional attribution of the values of caring and nurturing to women results in the stereotypical image of women as 'natural caregivers' (Miers, 2002). Tronto (1993) refers to this framing of care as 'women's morality' and warns that it turns care into a 'parochial concern of women' instead of 'a central concern of human life' (Tronto, 1993, p 180). In the account of care presented in this chapter the focus is on care for people living with AIDS in parts of sub-Saharan Africa with a high prevalence of HIV and AIDS. Even though the impacts of AIDS manifest themselves in different ways, prolonged and erratic care needs are a common feature. Care is provided mainly in the home and largely by women. At first glance, this may be viewed as just another case of women's morality. However, in this chapter I shall present evidence indicating that women's care for people living with AIDS also empowers them. This could encroach on the patriarchal order, turning care into a societal concern rather than only a parochial concern of women.

Within sub-Saharan Africa, there are substantial differences in HIV prevalence between countries. In West Africa prevalence is lowest, in southern Africa highest. Throughout the entire region female HIV prevalence rates are twice those of men (UNFPA, 2011, pp 112–14). This chapter focuses on evidence from South Africa, Tanzania and Zimbabwe. In Tanzania, for example, from 2000 onwards, female AIDS deaths consistently outnumber male AIDS deaths (Tanzania Country Report, 2012, p 11). As Barnett (2006, p 345) observes: 'In mature epidemics women are affected by HIV/AIDS more than men.'

He warns that 'assumptions about the availability of women's labor and skills for household and farm work may not hold in the future'.

Barnett's warning also applies to women's availability as care givers. Overwhelmingly, women bear the brunt of the burden of caring for persons suffering from AIDS, and communities and governments depend on their doing so (Makina, 2009). In Africa, apart from the role of medical professionals in antiretroviral treatment or crisis mitigation, care for people living with AIDS (including palliative care) is provided mainly by women in the home. In a survey on time use it was found that in Tanzania women bear the main burden of 'care of persons' in 84% of the cases involving 'active care'. The analysis distinguishes between a broader measure of 'care of persons' and a narrower measure of 'active care'. The latter excludes supervision of those needing care and travel related to care, both of which are regarded as 'passive care' (Budlender, 2010a, p 59). In a similar survey in South Africa, half of the 'already limited time' men spend on care is for 'passive care' (Budlender, 2010b, p 84). But since surveys like these are scarce, most of the evidence on women's role in care comes from micro-level studies. In a study about home-based care in KwaZulu-Natal, South Africa, for example, the team tried to find as many male care givers as possible, but only two could be found to include in the sample of 41 care givers (Akintola, 2006). Of the 14 care arrangements for people living with AIDS documented by Du Preez (2011, pp 133–5), 12 involved female care givers (10 family members and 2 neighbours). Several studies (Akintola, 2006; Nombo, 2007; Paradza, 2010; Du Preez, 2011) reveal the absence of men in AIDS-afflicted, *de facto* women-headed households. Akintola (2006, p 241) notes that 'abandonment of partners emerged as a subtle but effective and pervasive way of avoiding caring roles'.

As Peacock and Weston (2008, p 9) put it, 'gender identities and particular constructions of masculinity compound and contribute to the structural and political causes of the unfair and debilitating burden of care provided by women – especially in the context of HIV and AIDS'. As an important cause they mention the erosion of the public sector in Africa. This is a significant contextual factor when viewing care practice from an ethics-of-care perspective, because it comes down to the public sector relinquishing its care responsibilities. Other causes they mention, like the displacement of care into the household and onto women and girls, as well as the inertia of governments, are linked to this factor. To redress the situation, they propose a multi-pronged approach to increase men's share of the care burden, referring to interventions that were effective in transforming harmful gender attitudes and behaviour. However, here I want to take the issue further than the gender imbalance in care giving and its causes. Using findings of recent empirical research and looking at them from a different angle, I intend to elicit trends and patterns that – in my view – are part of a picture that has the contours of a matriarchy of care. Du Preez (2011) has already referred to the matrifocal nature of care and to matrilineality entering the patrilineal homestead in KwaZulu-Natal, South Africa, both of which can be seen as constituting components of a matriarchy of care.

Concepts and data

In line with the emergent paradigm based on the work by Joan Tronto (1993) and others, I see care as an ideologically and morally underpinned evolving social practice and, in agreement with Mol (2008), not as a commodity exchanged in transactions between care givers and care receivers. Informal care is based on pre-existing social relationships, develops as a process and is shaped by the social networks of care givers and care receivers (Ferlander, 2007) and by ideological notions about good care. Care provision is part of the moral economy of households that have to make available and allocate the resources for it (Niehof, 2004). Households operate in political economies, whether neoliberal or developing economies, in many of which care work tends to be undervalued, underpaid and mostly left to women (Tronto, 1993; Kittay, 2001a; Razavi, 2007; Makina, 2009).

Care is a gendered social practice. As Connell (2012, p 1677) stipulates in a review of policy documents and theoretical approaches, care practices are not random but 'occur in a dense and active social tissue of institutions and sites'. Care is also part of everyday domestic production (Niehof, 2004; Barnes, 2012a). As such, it is subject to routines. But 'routines are interesting because their seeming insignificance or invisibility may hide questions of power, freedom and control' (Ehn and Löfgren, 2009, p 99). Responding to evolving care needs necessitates changes of routine, confronting the actors concerned with new challenges. This could entail shifts in the gender balance, possibly resulting in the empowerment of women care givers. Therefore, I will align the presentation and discussion of the empirical evidence along the axes of care as practice and care as power.

For the empirical evidence I will especially draw on cases from research conducted in rural KwaZulu-Natal, South Africa (Du Preez and Niehof, 2008; Du Preez and Niehof, 2010; Du Preez, 2011), Tanzania (Nombo, 2007; Nombo and Niehof, 2008; Nombo, 2010) and Zimbabwe (Paradza, 2010). The African scholars were all participants in the AWLAE Project,[1] in which I was involved as a project coordinator and academic supervisor. I personally visited the field sites in Tanzania and South Africa. Common features of the areas where the fieldwork was done are: high HIV prevalence, high levels of (male) labour migration and population mobility, traditionally patrilineal kinship and patriarchal culture, and rural poverty. Rural KwaZulu-Natal has a long history of male labour migration but the patrilineal homestead has always been the mainstay of patriarchal Zulu culture (Mtshali, 2002). The spread of HIV and AIDS gave rise to reverse migration flows of men who return to their rural homesteads because they are sick and in need of care. The increasing numbers of people living with AIDS in rural areas led to people moving in and out of homesteads to provide or receive care (Du Preez and Niehof, 2010). Nombo's research site in Tanzania is an area where for decades the sugar plantation has attracted male migrant labour. This caused an increase of casual and transactional sex, high HIV prevalence, ethnic diversity and declining social cohesion. In conjunction with poverty and food insecurity, this led to a proliferation of witchcraft accusations and the deterioration of community structures (Nombo, 2007). In Zimbabwe, Paradza (2010) did her research in an area that originally was under patrilineal land tenure. Land distribution policies, economic crisis, structural adjustment, HIV/AIDS-induced population movement and changing rural–urban resource flows resulted in unstable local livelihoods and general uncertainty. In this situation, women and their children can no longer count on being provided for and have to fend for themselves; some of the women described by Paradza (2010) move frequently to find a place where they can access land to live and grow food crops for themselves and their children. These are the settings for which I will highlight women's caring roles and show how these have led to the emergence of what I call a matriarchy of care.

Care as practice

Tronto's vision of care as a 'life-sustaining web' (1993, p 103) is particularly applicable to home care for persons living with AIDS in sub-Saharan Africa. Without the life-sustaining web provided by their care givers, such people would live shorter lives, suffer more and die miserably.

Tronto (1993) distinguished four phases of care: caring about, taking care of, care giving and care receiving, which should all be part of a well-integrated process. This framework was applied in research on care for people living with AIDS in rural KwaZulu-Natal (Du Preez and Niehof, 2008; Du Preez, 2011). It was found that (mostly female) family members, neighbours and community health workers were alert to the care needs of persons living with AIDS in their environment and of indirectly affected community members like orphans (phase 1). They would then try to make suitable care arrangements (phase 2), which could involve approaching others for help or moving the person needing care to the place of the care giver.

Care as practice is most visible in the third phase. Du Preez and Niehof (2008, p 96) list the following care-giving practices: taking the patient to a healthcare facility; basic nursing care; physical care (feeding, bathing, toilet use); assisting with collecting and taking medication; rehabilitative care; psycho-social and spiritual support (being a companion in dealing with nearing death); and household assistance (cleaning, cooking, laundry). Akintola (2006, p 240) lists: moral and spiritual support (praying together); basic nursing care (treating sores, turning bedridden patients, checking drug adherence); help with daily activities (feeding, bathing, going to the toilet, dressing); help with household chores. Some of the few male care givers involved left the nursing care for their wife to a female volunteer. In Zulu culture men should be cared for by their wives and, if single, by their mothers, but sick women should not be seen by men and should be cared for by other women (Hutchings and Buijs, 2005).

The phases of care are gendered because access to the resources and capabilities needed is unequal for men and women. This applies especially to phases two and three. 'Taking care of' requires access to external resources, which needs bridging and linking social capital (Ferlander, 2007). 'Care giving' can be sustained only by bonding social capital. Men often have more bridging and linking social capital than women (cf Molyneux, 2002), whereas women – whether culturally prescribed (women as 'kinkeepers') or as a consequence of their nurturing and caring duties – have to rely on the strong ties that are part of bonding social capital. The cases I discuss provide many examples of (female) relatives and close neighbours helping women care givers. Care duties are largely defined by cultural scripts that determine the appropriateness of men's and women's roles and activities in care (Miers, 2002), the case of Zulu culture (see above) providing a telling example. However, changing circumstances such as in a context of HIV and AIDS (Niehof, 2012) induce different practices that may lead to cultural and institutional change, which is the core of the argument I present.

Also relating to care as practice is that the hegemonic construction of care giving as women's work leads to under-exposure of the role of male care givers in marital relationships. Montgomery et al (2006, p 2414) found that Zulu men actually do more care work than they are given credit for in the way people talk about it. Based on a case in a totally different context (that of a Pakistani family in England, where the husband cared for his terminally ill wife), Chattoo and Ahmad (2008) plead for the male voice in caring to be represented on its own. Budlender (2010a, p 68) warns that 'broad statements that claim that women and girls do all the unpaid care work in the Tanzanian economy and society are untrue and not helpful for policy-making purposes'. Hence, even though the share of men in care giving may be small, its visibility is obstructed by the societal framing of care as 'women's morality'.

A last note on the phases of care as practice concerns the relations between and the sequence of the phases. In the KwaZulu-Natal study (Du Preez, 2010) it was found that the phases can overlap and that a negative response of the care receiver to the provided care (phase 4) led to a change of care givers (phase 3) and to getting external help to make new care arrangements (phase 2). In short, the phases of care in fact together form multiple trajectories and their sequence can be reversed. With regard to AIDS in particular, this can be explained by the nature of the affliction. Care needs differ considerably according to its stage and the patient's use of antiretroviral drugs and prior general condition. This makes it difficult to anticipate care needs and provide for them when they change.

Care as power

In general, there is an inherent tension in the care giver–care receiver relationship that may even lead to hostility towards the care giver when the care receiver resents his/her dependence on the care giver. As Tronto (1993) noted, this would be less of an issue if we would all be more aware of our dependence on others throughout the life course. Because of AIDS, many women in Africa who could always depend on their adult children for support and care in their old age now find themselves caring for their sick and dying adult children and taking care of their orphaned grandchildren. This is experienced as a reversal of the 'natural' course of events (Nombo, 2007). Since HIV and AIDS especially affect adults in their prime, the epidemic upsets the dependency relations between the generations and deprives adult men and women of their agency and dignity. This makes the picture far more complex than that of a (temporary) power inequality between care givers and care receivers.

However, the power issues that are intrinsic to the caring relationship, the internal power dimension of care, are not the subject of this chapter. Instead, I focus on the external power dimension of care: the consequences of women's involvement in care for their position in the community and the possible long-term effects on society, which will be discussed in turn. I will here not go into the discourse on morality and power: why the one does not necessarily entail the other, and how women's morality is constructed in such a way that women do not derive power from it (see Tronto, 1993, on this point).

An analysis of five cases of care arrangements in rural KwaZulu-Natal (Du Preez and Niehof, 2010) yields a picture of a continuous reconfiguration of the living arrangements of persons suffering from AIDS or caring for people living with AIDS and of children of affected mothers. Regarding the latter, Budlender (2010b, p 70) also observed the frequent separation of parents and children in South Africa. One case is about two orphaned boys living on their own in the homestead of their deceased parents. The other four cases show how women give care, take care of situations, decide on who is going to live where, take in foster children and try to get child support grants. The women involved, as care givers or care receivers, are related as sisters or are mother and daughter or aunt and niece. In six of the ten cases described elsewhere (Du Preez and Niehof, 2008, p 94–5), women design and implement the care arrangements. Four of them are household heads, and all of them become the primary care giver (all mother–daughter relationships). In one case the husband set up the care arrangement for his sick wife and had his daughter do the care giving. In a similar case a woman was cared for by her husband together with a neighbour and a health worker. Another sick woman lives on her own and is looked after by neighbours and the community volunteer. A very sick young man living on his own was cared for by his grandmother. When she passed away, care was taken over by neighbours and a health worker. The community volunteers and neighbours who feature in the cases are all female.

The situation in Mkamba, Tanzania (Nombo, 2007) differs from that in rural KwaZulu-Natal in the virtual lack of support by relatives and neighbours. As a consequence of the area's history (discussed earlier), neighbours are not trusted and kinship networks have fallen apart. Nombo (2007, pp 129, 135, 145, 159) describes several situations in detail. The cases make clear that also in Mkamba it is women who care for their adult children suffering from AIDS and their orphaned grandchildren, even though they hardly have the means to do so. They take their sick son, daughter or sister into their home and try to generate some income to pay for the increased household expenses. They also try to mobilise financial support from an absent husband, a son(-in-law) or daughter who is not ill, or another relative, but only occasionally manage to get some. The support networks have contracted and some of the husbands have returned to their area of origin, leaving the women to take care of themselves and their dependants.

Paradza (2010) describes 22 units of single women with their children, which she calls hearth-holds: 'female-directed social units of consumption and production structured on the child–mother bond' (Paradza, 2010, p 79). In the literature these would be mostly classed as women-headed households, a term Paradza does not like because it implicitly makes the neoliberal male-headed household the standard of domestic organisation. Adult children live with their mother because of marital breakdown, unemployment or illness. Twenty-two hearth-holds are categorised according to their vulnerability status in terms of income and assets. Of these, 14 are vulnerable (Paradza, 2010, p 83). Seven of them are hosting ill adult children, the other seven have young children to care for. One hearth-hold, of which all members were ill, had fallen apart. Although Paradza selected these units purposively because they were headed by women, they are by no means rare cases. Because of Zimbabwe's recent history (see above), marriages tend to be unstable and, with the spread of HIV/AIDS, the probability of early widowhood is increased. The cases reveal women's agency in trying to secure access to land for residence and livelihood, in finding cash through income-earning activities or transfers (from the church, the community or family) and in taking care of their children, whether young or adult but ill. In one case, the mother, herself in ill health, was unable to cope and decided to send her children back to her ex-husband's homestead. Paradza (2010, p 88) sees this as 'some of the desperate choices that hearth-holds afflicted by AIDS and poverty have to make'.

The evidence presented above shows women as the pivotal actors in the care for AIDS patients and in the households directly or indirectly (fostering orphans) affected by AIDS. They not only do the care work but are instrumental in setting up and implementing care arrangements, across the boundaries of their own household and homestead if necessary and using bridging and linking social capital. The first is revealed in mobilising the support of health workers and church people, the second in accessing state child grants. While doing the care work as primary care givers can be another example of women's morality, arranging care and enlisting external support requires that women's authority in this is accepted and that they can yield a certain measure of power over others to comply. This I call the matriarchy of care.

The situation in KwaZulu-Natal differs from that in the other two cases in the level of support that women can claim and receive from the state and community health workers. The matriarchy of care is revealed by women's setting up care arrangements and securing the help of other household members, neighbours, relatives and health workers. They decide who is living where, while such decisions always were the prerogative of the male head of the homestead. The homestead as the embodiment of patrilineal kinship, virilocal residence and patriarchal culture (Mtshali, 2002) is changing into a site where not just providing for daily needs but, additionally, meeting the care needs generated by the AIDS epidemic has become a major concern. In this context, it is women who are taking the lead.

The matriarchal character of care is enforced by the central role of the mother–daughter relationship in care provision as well as by the importance of the support of maternal, female relatives. In this way, there also is a matrilineal side to care provision, as Du Preez (2011) noted. In an article on mother–daughter relationships following a health crisis (in the United States), the author speaks about 'evolving matriarchs', where mothers share with their daughters their ideas about inner strength and how to act upon these, in this way empowering their daughters (Shawler, 2007, p 844). More research would be needed to see how in the African HIV and AIDS context the care shared between mothers and daughters affects the gender notions and values in patriarchal cultures.

Conclusion

In the domain of food, similar questions as those for the domain of care have been raised about women's role and empowerment. The debate oscillates between the power of women as gatekeepers who control the food flows into their households on the one hand, and food work as reinforcing women's containment and subordination on the other (Allen and Sachs, 2012). Neither notion should be unthinkingly applied to the African context. Researching sex, food and power in Mozambique, Arnfred (2007, pp 148–9) found food to be 'a female domain and a basis for female authority'. The older women reign over the granaries and for all women cooking is 'a privilege and a pride'. In the same vein, the notion of care as 'a parochial concern of women' (Tronto, 1993, p 180) does not seem to apply to the African HIV and AIDS context, where care is the lifeline of the affected households and communities. Women's responsibilities for arranging care and finding support confer authority and express women's decision-making power. When this is the case, I think it is appropriate to speak of a matriarchy of care.

However, this is not the whole story. The evidence shows as well that because care is also practice, the resources have to be available to carry it out. The cases in Tanzania and Zimbabwe, in particular, also present women who do not have the means to make the arrangements work and are hardly able to enlist the support of others. Some of them become trapped in caring relationships that they feel as morally theirs but in which they neither have the material resources to provide good care nor the kind of social capital needed for securing assistance (Nombo and Niehof, 2008).

When the matriarchs of care are in control but in fact are empty handed, they will lose the authority vested in them and will succumb to the burden of their care responsibilities. In such a situation, care givers and care receivers are equally victims of poverty and inert governments, and lack voice to change that. This is an issue of social justice. Following a capabilities approach, policies should be geared towards 'what people are actually able to do and to be' (Nussbaum, 2003, p 39). Therefore, instead of being seen only as pitiable and overburdened, the women care givers should be credited for being the pivotal actors in the provision of AIDS care and for taking the responsibility to arrange care for AIDS patients and AIDS orphans. To enable them to perform these roles, governments should make an effort to make the necessary resources available and to increase access to antiretroviral treatment. In this regard, Tronto's fifth phase of 'caring with' (Tronto, 2013, p 22) applies. Kittay (2001a) argues that care giving (or 'dependency work' as she calls it) should be seen as part of citizenship and that the care giver also deserves care when needed. This refutes a narrow dyadic notion of reciprocity and, instead, pictures networks of reciprocal relationships embedded in a 'social responsibility for care' (Kittay, 2001a, p 536). If government policies and community politics were inspired by such a vision, in the provision of AIDS care women would be entitled to and receive government assistance and male support without having to sacrifice their authority and dignity.

The last point relates to the influence of the matriarchy of care on wider societal structures. For several reasons the AIDS epidemic is accelerating processes of social change in sub-Saharan Africa (Niehof, 2012). Also care as practice will incrementally induce social and cultural change, because even though care labour is largely part of household routines, routines can have a 'subversive potential'. Seemingly repetitive acts in everyday life may in fact 'produce small and successive changes, hardly perceived, but possibly important in the long run' (Ehn and Löfgren, 2009, p 111). I think this is happening, as the examples of women taking decisions about living arrangements and approaching non-kin for support show. Previously, such matters would be in the hands of men. Gradual change like this is compounded by the necessity of rethinking and adapting routines because of the prolonged and erratic nature of AIDS-related illness and because of the increasing numbers of afflicted women. Together these processes will impinge on and alter the gendered distribution of work, authority and power. Such processes engender social change through a mechanism that Giddens (1996) called structuration. Also, because the private–public boundary in most African societies is rather fluid and not much of a 'moral boundary' (cf. Tronto, 1993), practical and ideological change are spreading from the domestic domain to local communities and society at large.

Note

[1]   In the AWLAE Project, 20 women from 11 African countries did their PhD studies at Wageningen University on impacts of HIV and AIDS on women's roles in food and livelihood systems in sub-Saharan Africa.

TWELVE

HIV care and interdependence in Tanzania and Uganda

Ruth Evans and Agnes Atim

Introduction

The principle of 'Greater Involvement of People Living with or Affected by HIV/AIDS (PLHA)' declared at the 1994 Paris AIDS Summit provided widespread international commitment (in rhetoric at least) to the participation of people living with HIV in tackling the epidemic at all levels. Organisations and networks of PHLA have grown rapidly in eastern and southern Africa in recent years in order to campaign for their rights to health. Research in Tanzania and Namibia has revealed that care is often a two-way process of both giving and receiving care, based on reciprocal, interdependent relations between PLHA and family members (Evans and Thomas, 2009). PLHA may provide home-based care for partners, children, other family members and peers with HIV, as well as receiving care themselves. Such interdependent caring relations blur conventional boundaries and assumptions about the needs and interests of 'care givers' and 'care recipients', while simultaneously revealing interconnected dependencies and power inequalities at a range of spatial scales.

This chapter adopts an ethics of care perspective to explore PLHA's caring relations and participation within families and communities in Tanzania and Uganda and draws partly on ideas discussed in Evans and Atim (2011). We discuss the findings of three qualitative studies. The first two studies (conducted by Ruth Evans) focused on children's caring roles in families affected by HIV; the first was based on interviews with 20 mothers/female relatives living with HIV, 22 young people who cared for them and 13 non-governmental organisation (NGO) workers in rural and urban areas of Tanzania. This was part of a larger study funded by the UK Economic and Social Research Council that investigated the experiences, needs and resilience of children caring for parents and relatives with HIV in Tanzania and the UK (see Evans and Becker, 2009 for further information). The second study was focused on sibling care giving in child- and youth-headed households in Tanzania and Uganda, based on interviews, focus groups and participatory workshops with a total of 73 participants, comprising 17 orphaned children and young people who were caring for their siblings, 17 of their younger siblings and 25 NGO workers and 14 community members. This study was funded by the University of Reading and the Royal Geographical Society (with the Institute of British Geographers) (see Evans, 2011; 2012 for further information). The third study was based on doctoral research (conducted by Agnes Atim, part-funded by a University of Reading doctoral studentship) with a total of 80 participants, comprising interviews and focus groups with 18 men and 62 women living with HIV and 17 professionals in rural areas of Northern Uganda.In this chapter, we first give an overview of our theoretical approach. We then discuss how children and young people, who are often regarded as 'dependants', and women living with HIV, who are usually constructed as 'care recipients' or 'service users', play crucial roles in providing mutual emotional support and physical care within the family and community in Tanzania and Uganda. We then explore the roles of PLHA in peer support, care giving and healthcare delivery in East Africa. Several benefits of the participation of 'service users' are identified, alongside the challenges and constraints of achieving meaningful participation of PLHA in strategic decision-making processes.

Theorising interdependent caring relations

Disability theorists and feminists have highlighted the problematic nature of conventional notions of 'care', 'dependency' and 'autonomy' that establish a fixed binary opposition between the roles of care giver and care receiver (Morris, 1991; Shakespeare, 1993). Researchers have recognised that caring relationships are rarely simply a one-way process of 'giving' by one person to another, but rather are characterised by reciprocity and interdependence between the person living with illness or disability and the 'carer' (Evans and Becker, 2009). Tronto's (1993) and Sevenhuijsen's (1998) ethics of care recognise the interdependence and interconnectedness of human relations, responsibilities and practices of care. Caring is valued as a daily practice in everyone's lives and it is acknowledged that there is no absolute or fixed division of roles between care giver and care receiver.

Work on emotional geographies recognises the ways that people living with illness or disability and their carers negotiate complex emotions (Davidson and Milligan, 2004; Evans and Thomas, 2009). Bondi suggests that the notion of 'empathic understanding' enables care givers to 'imaginatively identify with care-recipients without confusing their own feelings with those they imagine to be felt by care-recipients. It is equally what enables care-recipients to imagine what it might be like for care-givers to do what they do' (2008, p 260). She explains that this fosters good communication between care givers and care receivers, which helps to ensure that care needs have been met, corresponding to Tronto's ethical value of 'responsiveness'.

Fine and Glendinning's (2005) understanding of 'relational autonomy' (Mackenzie and Stoljar, 2000) and Kittay's (2002b) theorisation of the power relations imbued in notions of 'care' and 'dependency' are also helpful in exploring the participation of PLHA in care, support and advocacy at local, national and global levels. Fine and Glendinning (2005) suggest that 'independence' can be conceptualised as 'relational autonomy'; power should not only be regarded as negative but, rather, can be understood as 'capability', 'as a form of empowerment – "power to" not "power over"'(p 616). Empowerment is understood in terms of a person's agency and their capacity to do or affect something and 'make a difference'. Kittay (2002b) distinguishes between 'inequality of power' and the 'exercise of domination' in care giving; inequalities of power do not mean that abuse is inherent in the caring relationship, which is ideally based on mutual trust and responsibility. Domination, however, represents a breakdown of this mutual trust by either the worker (the paid or unpaid care giver) or the charge (the care recipient) (Fine and Glendinning, 2005, p 613).

Kittay (2002b) suggests that a second level of dependency is based on the reliance of the charge and the dependency worker on 'the provider', who controls the resources needed to provide care and creates the conditions which devalue 'dependency work'. The state may be regarded as the provider, but in Tanzania, Uganda and other low-income countries in the global South, state welfare support is virtually non-existent and health systems are severely constrained, especially in post-conflict settings. In this context, the notion of a provider could also encompass donor aid and global institutions and funding streams such as the US President's Emergency Fund for AIDS Relief and the Global Fund to fight AIDS, tuberculosis and malaria. The second level of dependency is thus characterised by power inequalities at the global and national scales that prevent equal access to healthcare and constrain the ability of governments and healthcare providers to provide support for all those who require assistance, as well as by social arrangements at the local level (Evans and Atim, 2011). This highlights the need to contextualise caring relations and institutions at multiple, interconnected scales, as we seek to do in this chapter.

Interdependent caring relations within families

Research in Eastern and Southern Africa has revealed that care is often characterised by strong emotional connections between PLHA and those who care for them (Chimwaza and Watkins, 2004; Evans and Thomas, 2009). In the sibling care-giving research, many young people heading households share the domestic and care work with their siblings, developing reciprocal relations of care and support within the home that can accommodate their schooling and livelihood activities. Rickson (aged 19), who was caring for two younger siblings, commented:

> "Since I stay with my two siblings, we have shifts. If I have time today I cook, so that s/he can be able to study. If it is tomorrow, I can study when s/he is cooking. The other day I study and s/he cooks. Just like that. So, we change shifts."

Many mothers with HIV and children caring for them in Tanzania reported that they had close, loving relationships and understood each other well. Children played a key role in providing emotional support to their mothers, siblings and other relatives living with HIV. Despite mothers' illness and the emotional support children provided, however, most children said that they turned to their mother for advice, guidance and support. Mothers/adult relatives with HIV retained their usual position of authority and responsibility for decision making within the household, despite sometimes being nursed in bed for several months. The continued parenting role of mothers refutes negative assumptions about the competence of parents living with HIV to provide good care for their children (Evans and Atim, 2011).

Some mothers' and young people's narratives demonstrate a strong sense of empathy and understanding of the emotional pressures the other person in the caring relationship may be experiencing. Husna, a mother with HIV, reflected on why Juliette (aged 20) had greater caring responsibilities than her other daughters: "I feel she is the one who understands my situation better. She is very compassionate. It is obvious that she really depends on me and I on her." Juliette, who was studying at a teacher training college away from home during term time, commented on the emotional dimensions of her caring responsibilities:

"Whenever I get a letter from home saying she is very poorly, I can't concentrate at all. I am filled with thoughts like what would happen to us if she died. I have my younger sisters, I would be the one to look after for them. It is better when she is alive, I feel as though she is helping me in a way because she inspires me with hope. I feel very much at peace seeing her alive."

Such close emotional connections within caring relationships help to ensure that care is based on (among others) the ethical value of 'responsiveness' (Tronto, 1993). These connections highlight the complexity of caring relations within families and reveal fluidity between the roles of care givers and care recipients.

Despite tensions in some families, many young people felt that their caring role had made them 'stronger' and more emotionally mature (Evans, 2013). The life-limiting nature of their parent's illness and the vulnerability of their younger siblings, however, limited the reciprocity of emotional support. Young people caring for parents with HIV felt that they needed to regulate and manage their emotions so as to avoid their parent becoming worried or stressed, as they knew this could make their illness worse (Evans and Thomas, 2009). Furthermore, young people heading households in Tanzania and Uganda did not feel that they could turn to their younger siblings for emotional support and several lacked opportunities to share their feelings with others. In workshops in Tanzania, siblings identified loneliness and the need to suppress their feelings as some of the worst aspects of heading the household: "I feel lonely when I see my friends being brought up by their parents," and "I'm forced to be happy all the time, even though I'm sad". While several siblings were proud of their role heading the household, they expressed ambivalence about having to take on a parenting role for their siblings while they still considered themselves to be a young person (Evans, 2013).

In Tanzania, many mothers with HIV were concerned about how caring affected their children's emotional well-being. Husna said of Juliette's caring responsibilities:

"She has a big burden on her young shoulders. I sometimes feel she is overwhelmed by worry. She thinks a lot about me and I think she dreads the day I will die because she will have to provide for her younger sisters. [...] I am sad but I have no choice. I feel sorry for her because I feel she is carrying the burden of someone else's responsibility, but that someone else isn't there."

Juliette perceived her caring responsibilities as 'daunting' at times, but felt a moral obligation to support her mother, since their relatives stigmatised the family and they lacked alternative sources of support: "The responsibilities are many and I am still young. At times it is daunting. But there is no one else to help so I have to do it".

Similarly, some of the young people heading households commented on the loneliness and emotionally demanding nature of the care they provided for younger siblings:

> "When I have all these responsibilities at home, firstly, I think of my parents. When I think about my parents, I get pain in my heart. Therefore when I have these negative thought, I reach a point of losing hope. I say to myself 'why am I here just alone?' However, since [NGO] are teaching us about perseverance, how can we get out of this situation, I persevere because I am not alone." (Hamisa, young woman aged 19, caring for her young cousin in Tanzania)

Thus, despite the development of interdependent, reciprocal caring relations, mutual trust and responsibility within families affected by HIV, some mothers and young people simultaneously perceived care as a 'burden' which could have negative physical, emotional and educational impacts on young people. The 'diminished autonomy' of care givers here can be regarded as a consequence of a lack of alternative co-resident care givers, the limited formal safety nets available to families affected by HIV in East Africa and global power inequalities that limit the capacity of the 'provider', creating a secondary level of dependency (Kittay, 2002b).

Peer support, care giving and the participation of PLHA 'service users' in healthcare

Opportunities for marginalised groups to meet, share experiences and develop peer support in safe spaces may be empowering for individuals. Peer support among those who identify with a particular health identity is often focused on coming to terms with the diagnosis, sharing embodied experiences and learning about biomedical health and treatment issues associated with their condition (Beckmann and Bujra, 2010). Many women in Tanzania regularly attended peer support groups, which they felt provided opportunities for women to share experiences and give informal advice about HIV-related issues, including adherence to treatment, nutrition and gaining access to informal material support. Similarly, orphaned young people caring for their siblings in Tanzania, who received support from an NGO, commented on the importance of peer support in helping them to cope with the loss of their parents and in continuing in their caring roles:

> "I felt very bad because losing both parents, I was sad for about four months. I was thinking of my parents. But I had to get used and leave it, and be like others, because others lose their parents as well. So we were exchanging ideas with other youths like me who have lost their parents, on how to live, we exchanged ideas and [...] we got used to it." (Rickson, aged 19, caring for two younger siblings in Tanzania)

Peer support can also foster collective mobilisation and action to challenge discrimination and barriers to participation. Indeed, the research from Tanzania suggests that sustained youth-led community action helped to reduce the stigma and harassment that orphaned youth experienced in Kagera region, north-western Tanzania (Clacherty and Donald, 2006; Madoerin, 2008).

PLHA in Uganda engaged in home-based care from the peak of the epidemic in the early 1990s in order to reduce barriers to care, provide peer support and bring healthcare to those who were unable to travel to a clinic. PLHA played a crucial role in providing comprehensive non-clinical nursing, palliative, psycho-social and spiritual care to their peers. With the scale-up of antiretroviral therapy (ART, often referred to as ARVs) from the mid-2000s onwards, many PLHA became home-based care givers and community support agents based in health facilities in order to provide support in adherence to treatment (Cataldo et al, 2008). Such community support roles help to reduce the likelihood of PLHA who have tested positive subsequently failing to return to health facilities to receive treatment and other services. The greater participation of PLHA in healthcare provision was largely instigated as a means of addressing the limited access to HIV information, services and care available to PLHA in Uganda at the time.

The research suggests that peer-led care and support activities became a key way for PLHA to participate in healthcare service provision, in recognition of each other's common vulnerabilities and interdependence. Participants involved in healthcare delivery reported that they were motivated by their own experiences of living with HIV and their wish to increase access to healthcare services. For example, Eunice's experiences of gaining access to treatment when she most needed it inspired her to 'save other lives' by enabling other PLHA to access treatment:

> "When I tested positive in 1993, I knew that was the end of my life. By then drugs were very expensive that I couldn't afford, my husband had just died and I was pregnant. There were no PMTCT [Prevention of Mother-to-Child-Transmission of HIV] programmes yet at that time, my daughter got infected and later died when she was four. My CD4[1] went down to 21 at the time government started providing free ARV in 2002 and I was the first client to register to get ARV from Lira hospital. Since then I decided to do all I can to save lives and stop other children and adults from dying as my husband and child did."

Healthcare providers and policy makers in Uganda, as well as care recipients and care givers, saw PLHA's involvement in healthcare as necessary to increase access to care for all those who needed it. Indeed, involvement by service users in the delivery of healthcare and support services may help to reduce the burden of care on dysfunctional healthcare systems in post-conflict, resource-constrained settings, such as in Northern Uganda. The research suggests that PLHA have played an important role in shifting the health system paradigm from service delivery 'for the community' to 'by the community' (Sarkar, 2010, p 3). The roles PLHA undertook included: acting as service delivery agents and points of contact at the community level; providing care and support services; working alongside health workers in health facilities; and client referral, tracking and follow-up to increase access to health services. PLHA also coordinated and facilitated linkages between households, the community, health facilities, NGOs, policy makers and development partners.

The research suggests that PLHA's involvement in delivering HIV prevention, treatment, care and support services led to increased uptake of HIV services and a reduction in stigma in the study locations. Increased participation of PLHA in providing care and support can also directly benefit PLHA and care givers, as well as healthcare providers. As we found in the research on young people's caring roles in families affected by HIV, the caring relations that developed between PLHA in Uganda enhanced emotional ties and were based on mutual trust and the ethical values of 'empathic understanding' and 'responsiveness'. John, for example, commented on the strong sense of empathy and understanding of the needs of PLHA that he experienced by his peers' providing him with home-based care in the context of high levels of stigma and discrimination:

> "I am here today because of this man [a fellow participant in the focus group]. He broke into the house, where my family had locked me up for days, so that nobody could see me because it would bring shame to the family. He counselled me, carried me on his bicycle to hospital and even attended to me in the hospital, until I could stand up and walk again. I will do anything to help a fellow PLHA because of what he did to me."

Service users' 'empathic understanding' of the needs of their peers helped to ensure that PLHA care and support was 'people-centred' and responsive to their needs, which is especially important in post-conflict settings, where people feel they have lost everything. As Bella pointed out:

> "I visit clients in their homes, bath, wash their clothes, collect water, cook, put food on the table and talk to them especially for bedridden clients. This is the service one needs most when bedridden. I was cared for and supported a lot by peers when I was bedridden. I know how valuable it was in my life, that is why I feel I should provide care to someone who needs it."

Despite these benefits of participation, the increased involvement of service users in delivering healthcare and support services can also be seen as fulfilling neoliberal donor-driven agendas of promoting participation, providing alternative service delivery and shifting responsibility for care from the state onto unpaid caregivers, who are mostly women and girls (Ogden et al, 2006; McIlwaine, 2007). This raises the question of the role of the state and global institutions and donors, and whether PLHA, the majority of whom are unpaid volunteers, should be expected to take on such healthcare delivery and care and support roles when they are already struggling to provide for their own households. Indeed, the detrimental impact of PLHA's care-giving roles on their own livelihoods was highlighted as a key issue by women in Uganda. As a result of feedback discussions with participants, Agnes (second author) helped the women to establish a 'Care for the Carers' organisation that secured donor funding to support the agricultural livelihoods of 220 care givers living with HIV in Northern Uganda.

The wider question remains, however, of whether, by PLHA adopting these roles in HIV care and support and healthcare delivery, the state, global institutions and donors are absolved from having to train and pay healthcare professionals to provide these services. An ethic-of-care perspective offers a political argument for the values of care to represent the starting point for the development of social policies and interventions in all sectors and social institutions, including healthcare, social care, community development and family practices (Sevenhuijsen, 2000; Barnes, 2006). Such a political argument for care would reimagine democratic life and envision a rather different 'caring democracy' (Tronto, 2013) than the existing market-driven reliance on PLHA volunteers to provide unpaid healthcare services and to make up for gaps in funding, human resources and service provision in the global South.

Furthermore, the research found that PLHA's participation in healthcare service delivery in Uganda was highly gendered and often reinforced conventional gender roles and norms. Home-based care tasks that involved physical and emotional labour, such as bathing, personal care, domestic chores and providing counselling and psycho-social dimensions of support, were often constructed as 'women's work'. Men's involvement in healthcare was usually limited to conventional male-dominated roles, such as building a house for a weak PLHA in the community or giving health talks with fellow men in places where men usually socialise. As a man living with HIV explained, "In my home I don't cook, I don't collect water or sweep the house, how do you expect me to take care of a bedridden patient? What will people think about me doing a woman's work?" Men were also more likely than women to be involved in paid healthcare roles, such as working as expert clients, as health facility-based health educators, in village health teams and so on, which were associated with a higher status than home-based care and were rewarded through an income or a bicycle. Dominant gender norms could thus be reinforced through PLHA's increased participation in healthcare and peer support activities.

While our research suggests that developing peer support and living more positively with HIV was important in reducing isolation and may enhance PLHA's 'relational autonomy', it is unclear how this may translate into wider collective action and politicisation in campaigning and advocacy beyond the local level. Although peer support groups and peer-led home-based and clinic-based care and support activities were highly valued, they were not usually linked to national networks of PLHA or to transnational activism. Beckmann and Bujra (2010) found that access to antiretroviral therapy enabled PLHA in Tanzania to pass as 'normal' and conceal their illness from others. This may mean, however, that people no longer identify as PLHA and disengage from peer support and activist activities. Our research suggests that, despite the high level of involvement of PLHA in care and support activities at local level, their participation in HIV care and support decision-making processes, policy and advocacy at national and global scales has been limited to date.

Several advocacy initiatives are on-going to raise awareness of care givers' issues and the burden of care on women in the context of HIV. Agnes (the second author), has participated in several global forums on HIV care and support, including at the United Nations General Assembly Special Session meetings on HIV and AIDS in New York, in recent years. A global Caregivers Action Network was established by key stakeholders in 2009 and Agnes established the Caregivers Action Network Africa at the 2012 International AIDS Conference in Washington, DC in order to further develop policy, research and care givers' mobilisation in Africa.

A number of challenges to PLHA's participation in global and national policies and decision-making processes on HIV care and support, however, remain (Evans and Atim, 2011). The inclusion of the care and support of PLHA in the 2005 Universal Access to antiretroviral therapy targets and in the global care agenda of the 2009 United Nations Commission on the Status of Women were major steps forward in recognising the holistic needs of PLHA. In practice, however, medical treatment activities are much more visible and quantifiable and the achievement of measurable targets, such as universal antiretroviral therapy access targets and Millennium Development Goal 6, are considered a priority for governments, international donors and United Nations agencies. This has resulted in recent years in an overwhelming emphasis on the scaling-up of antiretroviral therapy in funding and programme responses, to the detriment of the care and support agenda. This has been accompanied by limited civil society advocacy on care and support issues, as compared with treatment activism. Weak global governance of HIV care and support activities, such as the lack of a powerful guiding institution at global level with clear responsibilities for care and support, has hindered implementation. Within the United Nations care and support is seen as a crossing-cutting issue with no single lead agency and no inter-agency task team responsible for care and support aspects of the HIV response.

Further challenges relate to perceptions and attitudes towards HIV and care. While increased access to antiretroviral therapy has led to a welcome reduction in AIDS-related mortality, and PLHA accessing treatment who have an adequate, nutritional diet are now able to lead relatively 'normal' lives, this has resulted in a strong perception that care and support services are no longer required. HIV is increasingly viewed as a chronic illness that can be effectively managed through bio-medical intervention, rather than as a terminal illness. Narrow understandings of care among policy makers and practitioners and the fact that most care givers are women and girls hinder the development of care services and support for PLHA. The lack of priority accorded to HIV care and support by healthcare institutions, policy makers and government reflects gendered assumptions about women's 'natural' (and hence unpaid) roles in caring for ill and disabled family members and the widespread devaluing of care due to its association with privacy, emotion and the 'othering' of those in need (Sevenhuijsen, 2000). Such perspectives conflict with a feminist ethic of care that recognises the importance of care for all human beings and values it as everyone's responsibility (Tronto, 1993; 2013). Finally, unequal gender and generational relations in many cultural contexts mean that the voices of women, girls and boys who are care givers and/or living with HIV are often marginalised in decision-making processes from the macro to the micro levels.

Conclusion

Our research in Tanzania and Uganda suggests that children and young people and women living with HIV, who are usually constructed as 'dependants', 'care recipients' or 'service users', play crucial roles in providing reciprocal emotional support, guidance, health and practical care for family members and peers living with HIV. Indeed, the two-way process of care giving and care receiving often led to close emotional ties, reciprocity, interdependence and a high level of responsiveness, challenging binary assumptions about the identities and practices of care givers and care receivers. The research also reveals, however, the intensity of intimate caring relations and problems of social isolation and inadequate resources facing families affected by HIV. This may cause tensions and contradictory feelings about a perceived burden of care that may be difficult to manage (Evans and Thomas, 2009). These conflicts can severely constrain care givers' ability to provide 'good care' (Tronto's, 1993), resulting in diminished autonomy for care givers and care recipients. This sense of 'diminished autonomy' (Fine and Glendinning, 2005) and the disempowerment of those involved in caring relationships is further compounded by the second level of dependency (Kittay, 2002b) related to inequalities in access to healthcare and welfare support at local, national and global scales.

Our research suggests, however, that peer support among families affected by HIV and the participation of PLHA in healthcare delivery and care giving in East Africa may have several benefits, including helping to promote empowerment and reduce feelings of dependency on family members, thereby alleviating potential tensions and emotional pressures within caring relations and the risk of 'domination' and abandonment (Kittay, 2002b). PLHA care givers in Uganda were motivated to provide the best care they could because they knew that they might develop such care needs themselves in future, thereby fostering an environment of 'reciprocal social co-operation' (Kittay, 2002b, p 271). Indeed, the research suggests that the participation of people living with HIV in healthcare provision, home-based care and peer support groups can enhance 'relational autonomy' for both care givers and care recipients, although such initiatives often play out in highly gendered ways. Gendered and generational power imbalances could be reinforced, as well as contested, through the care and peer support that children and PLHA provide.

The increased involvement of 'service users' in delivering healthcare and support services raises important questions about the role of the state, global institutions and donors, and whether the participation in healthcare of people living with HIV is merely fulfilling the neoliberal donor-driven agenda of providing alternative service delivery (McIlwaine, 2007) and shifting responsibility for care from the state onto unpaid caregivers, who are mostly women and girls. While PLHA are increasingly taking on crucial roles in HIV prevention, care and support within local communities in resource-constrained, post-conflict settings, such as in Northern Uganda, their participation in strategic decision-making processes at the national and global levels is limited. The research therefore highlights the need for an ethic of care that recognises and values women's, girls' and boys' care work, places the values of care at the centre of the development of health and social care policies and practices and addresses the structural inequalities and gendered power imbalances that restrict the participation of people living with HIV, especially care-giving women and girls, at local, national and global scales. As Tronto (2013, p 169) argues, this involves reimagining democratic life as on-going practices and institutions in which all citizens are engaged and 'presumes that relational selves, who need ongoing participation as both receivers and givers of care, will be central in making judgments about responsibility'.

Acknowledgements

We are grateful to all the participants in Tanzania and Uganda for sharing their experiences with us. We thank Sophie Bowlby and Sally Lloyd-Evans for their support and gratefully acknowledge the ESRC, Royal Geographical Society (with the Institute of British Geographers) and University of Reading for funding the research reported here. Agnes wishes to thank all the PLHA fraternity in Northern Uganda, particularly NACWOLA Lira; Agago and Lira Network of People Living with HIV; the Healthcare professionals, political leaders and NGO workers in Lira and Agago districts for their valuable information that made her research possible.

Note

1   CD4, also known as helper T-cells, act as a coordinator of the immune response in the body. HIV destroys infected CD4+ T-cells, leading to an overall weakening of the immune system and can also be indicative of the success or failure of antiretroviral therapy (WHO, 2014). In 2006, the World Health Organization recommended that the criteria for the initiation of antiretroviral therapy (ART) in adults in resource-limited settings is for ART to be considered when the CD4 cell count was between 200 and 350 and for those with less than 200 to be treated irrespective of the clinical stage of HIV-associate disease, since this is associated with a significant increase in opportunistic infections and death (WHO, 2006). These guidelines were revised upwards in 2010 to recommend that all adolescents and adults, including pregnant women, with HIV infection and CD4 counts of equal to or under 350 cells/mm^3, should start ART, regardless of the presence or absence of clinical symptoms. Those with severe or advanced clinical disease (WHO clinical stage 3 or 4) should start ART irrespective of their CD4 cell count (WHO, 2010).

THIRTEEN

Reciprocity and mutuality: people with learning disabilities as carers

Nicki Ward

Introduction

In the introduction to this collection we posed the question 'why now?' in relation to the salience of exploring and developing the feminist ethic of care. This chapter, while focused on carers who have a learning disability, is in many ways representative of wider demographic and policy shifts that have marked the delivery of social care in Western society since the 1980s. Improved healthcare means that families are living longer and are ageing together in ways that generate new and shifting relationships of care. At the same time, policies that have sought to enhance the rights and independence of people with learning disabilities have also contributed to new patterns of care. Disability activists have argued that those with disabilities are disempowered by relationships of care (Morris, 2004; Beckett, 2007). However, the social practices of care explored here suggest a more complicated picture that is illustrative of nested relationships of care (Barnes, Chapter Three in this volume) and suggestive of the need to adopt a post-structuralist understanding of power, positioning and multiple intersectional identities (Ward, N., Chapter Five in this volume).

Debates about the way that decisions made in the public sphere can impact on private lives are also significant here. Public and social policies and political decision making, as well as our social interactions, all impact on our daily lives and in this way the boundary between the public and the private can be seen as artificial (Tronto, 1993). For people with learning disabilities, because they are deemed vulnerable and in need of care and protection, their lives are, more than most, shaped and influenced by public policy. The experiences of carers with learning disabilities explicitly demonstrate the way that private relationships of care and support are impacted on by public discourses that contribute to the construction of them as (dis)abled as well as denoting how they are supported by public policy.

The practice of care is a social one through which moral considerations are expressed (Sevenhuijsen, 1998); it is not purely an emotional or intuitive response, but one that involves the person in actively thinking through and making judgements about the best thing to do in the situation and, as such, it is an expression of moral agency. These practices of care are variable, influenced by the different dynamics of caring relationships as well as the 'norms and rules' that define good care (Sevenhuijsen, 1998, p 22). Critical care ethics emphasise the importance of people's autobiographical experiences through which relationships, care and social connections can be interpreted as expressions of morality (Robinson, 1999, p 18). This is explored here from the perspective of people with learning disabilities who are carers, as reflected in their lived experiences. Drawing on a consultation that was conducted with carers with learning disabilities in England I will demonstrate the way that people with learning disabilities enact care ethics through their caring roles, while also exploring the barriers that they face in doing so. The consultation used a range of methods, including workshops, questionnaires and e-mail conversations, to gather information from carers with learning disabilities about their experiences; a total of 32 people shared experiences (Baker et al, 2012). The 19 people who participated in the workshops were aged between 20 and 70 and included 7 men and 12 women, one of whom was South Asian.

I begin by considering the concepts of reciprocity and mutuality, and the importance of these concepts to people with learning disabilities who are carers. The social practices of care are constructed and experienced discursively (Sevenhuijsen, 1998); for people with learning disabilities who are carers this has particular resonance in terms of the creation of visibility and invisibility and the extent to which their roles as carers are understood and supported. Following this I consider how the aspects of care ethics identified by Tronto – attentiveness, responsibility, competence, responsiveness (2013, pp 34–5) – enable reciprocity and mutuality and the extent to which, for carers with learning disabilities, the matrices of care within which they are involved enable them to fulfil their roles as care givers.

Mutuality and reciprocity

Being involved in a relationship of care – whether as care giver, care receiver or both – makes obvious the interdependence of human individuals and presents a challenge to the idea that people are or should be completely independent (Tronto, 1993, p 134). In this consultation it became apparent that people with learning disabilities were involved in successive multiple relationships of care within which they fulfilled the roles of both care giver and care receiver, often simultaneously. All of the people who participated in the workshops had at least one person in their life who was identified as their care giver and all had been care givers themselves. Nine of the workshop participants had had multiple caring roles throughout their lives and the people they had cared for included parents, grandparents, siblings, partners, friends and children. Three people indicated that they were currently caring for more than one person. It was also apparent that these relationships developed and changed over time – explicitly demonstrating the nested nature of mutual care relationships. People with learning disabilities who are carers are very clear about this. Perhaps because they have been positioned as care receivers for much of their lives they are able to identify the changes to these relationship patterns. This was most clearly expressed by one workshop participant who cared for his mother, when he noted: 'roles can be reversed, we look after each other now'. While our needs for care shift and change over time we all have inevitable dependencies (Kittay, 1999), such that our lives are embedded with relationships of care and dependency (Engster, 2005, p 61). It is this interdependency and interconnectedness that care ethics emphasises in the context of our mutual need for care. While this is widely acknowledged in discussion of care ethics in this chapter I am discussing a more explicit enactment of mutuality where people are fulfilling both care-giver and care-receiver roles at the same time. Mutual care is a notion that is gaining resonance in the UK in relation to people with learning disabilities as carers. Approximately 30% of people with learning disabilities live in residential care, while only 15% have their own homes; the remainder live predominantly with family carers (Emerson et al, 2005; DH, 2009). The increase in life expectancy, both for people with learning disabilities (DH, 2001b) and for the population more generally, means that many people are now living in ageing families (DH, 2009) with relatives who are themselves now in need of care. In many of these households people with learning disabilities are now involved in mutual caring relationships, still receiving care and support from their family members, but at the same time providing care for them in what can be seen as an explicit enactment of mutual interdependency.

For people with learning disabilities being a care giver provides an opportunity to demonstrate reciprocity and through this to adopt a valued social role more often denied to them. The concept of reciprocity is used not to represent the idea that people are 'trading favours' in a 'you scratch my back, I'll scratch yours' transaction; rather, I am suggesting that reciprocity should be recognised as necessary to supporting interdependence. Sevenhuijsen has argued elsewhere that trust is necessary to oil the wheels of care (1998). Here the argument is two-fold, firstly that reciprocity is important in nurturing and supporting mutual interdependence and secondly that opportunities to enact reciprocity through and within relationships of care are something that is recognised as a valued social role. In this way reciprocity of care is something that is important to people with learning disabilities who are carers (Ward, 2011; Baker et al, 2012). Engster (2005) highlights the importance of the reciprocal and mutual elements of care relationships. The need to care is, he suggests, driven by our own dependency and the knowledge that we both have been dependent and continue to be dependent upon others. For most of the carers with learning disabilities who shared their thoughts and experiences with us this was an important theme; they understand their roles now as being representative of mutual care and reciprocity and through this they gain self-esteem and an increased sense of their importance and worth within their relationships and within the wider world. It has been suggested that reciprocity is a concept that gains increasing resonance in the lives of older adults (Tanner, 2010; Lloyd et al, 2012), and it was through the mutual roles of care, often with older adults, that this became important for people with learning disabilities.

People with learning disabilities are one of the most excluded groups in UK society (Williams, 2009), and such exclusions encompass both material and discursive dimensions (Ward, 2009). The positioning of people with learning disabilities as vulnerable and in need of care and protection contributes to their becoming marginalised and excluded. One consequence of this is that their roles within society are not recognised and valued. In order for this situation to be addressed they have a need for recognition to alleviate the cultural and symbolic injustice that they face as a result of the inequitable social patterns of representation and non-recognition (Fraser, 1997). For Tronto (1993) a 'morally good person' is one who 'strives to meet the demands of caring that present themselves' (p 126). While carers with learning disabilities demonstrate their ability to do this, often on multiple occasions (Baker et al, 2012), they are rarely perceived as carers or credited with fulfilling this role (Holman et al, 2009). Exploring the experiences of people with learning disabilities who are carers enables us to see how they express the attributes of caring moral citizenship in their everyday lives, through mutual and reciprocal relationships of care.

A critical ethic of care understands care as an extremely complex, political act that requires those involved in it to be morally and cognitively engaged (Tronto, 1993, p 136; Sevenhuijsen, 1998, p 137). As noted above, people with learning disabilities who are carers are usually simultaneously care receivers and, as such, they are involved in complex networks of care involving paid care workers, families, friends and communities. In the section that follows I will consider how people with learning disabilities who are carers demonstrate their caring morality, while also considering the support they receive to enable them to do this within their networks of care. This is done by employing the dimensions of care identified and explicated by Tronto (1993), who suggests that care ethics is 'a habit of mind' that encapsulates four 'ethical elements of care: attentiveness, responsibility, competence and responsiveness' (p 127). The moral aspects of the care ethic need to be used in a way that acknowledges the context of the care process. In the next section these aspects will be explored in relation to the experiences of carers with learning disabilities and their networks of care.

Attentiveness: caring about

Attentiveness involves the capacity to notice the need for care; we cannot address the care needs of another person without this recognition. While this may seem like a simple act it requires our being able to consider the world from the perspective of another and it is therefore a 'moral achievement' (Tronto, 1993, p 127). Most people with learning disabilities have been positioned as a care receiver throughout their lives and this enables a person not only to 'see' the need for care but also to understand the importance of 'good care' (see also Fudge Schormans, Chapter Fourteen in this volume). In this sense people with learning disabilities can become particularly attuned to moral attentiveness because of their own experiences, thus evidencing the argument that caring practices can give rise to caring attitudes (Tronto, 2013, p 49).

For some people with learning disabilities the practices of care they have received have not always been positive and may even have been experienced as disempowering. This too has enhanced their understanding of what it means to be attentive to the needs of another. Those who responded to this consultation talked about knowing what good and bad care was and drew on their own learning and experiences of self-advocacy in order to fulfil their roles as care givers. So, for example, during a discussion about what it meant to be a carer one participant, who had had multiple caring roles in her life, suggested that it included 'visiting in hospitals and homes and *speaking up* when things are not right'.

In order for a care giver to be able to care well they need to be able to identify their own care needs and have these met (Tronto, 1993, p 131). This notion of 'caring for the carer' is one that has become embedded within UK policy, in both the work of statutory and non-statutory organisations (DH, 2010b; Carers Trust, 2014; Carers UK, 2014). The rights of carers to support have also been embedded in legislation and carers have a right to an assessment of their support needs under the Carers and Disabled Children Act 2000. Not only is attention to the care needs of care givers important, its absence can create barriers to 'being a carer'. While people with learning disabilities who are carers demonstrate their attentiveness to the needs of others, they also recognise the failure of others to be attentive to their needs as care givers. Caring for the carer to enable them to fulfil their caring roles requires being able to see and recognise the person traditionally seen as vulnerable and in need of care – the care receiver – as a potential and actual care giver. Tronto (1993), in discussing the work of Arendt on 'evil' notes that a failure to be attentive can come from ignorance, including the 'established habits of ignorance' (p 128). Policy discourse has traditionally constructed relationships of care as unidirectional, and within this people with learning disabilities are seen as the vulnerable partners and therefore the ones in need of care. This discourse renders people with learning disabilities who are carers invisible and is part of a process of non-recognition. Those who took part in the consultation consistently expressed frustration at this lack representation and the impact that it had on their caring roles. During discussion, carers with learning disabilities talked about the fact that policy makers thought that they could not be carers, noting 'but we are doing it, we are proving them wrong', and the overriding recommendation was that politicians needed to hear the voices of carers with learning disabilities and do something to support them.

A caring morality on the part of others was important in enabling or hampering the ability of people with learning disabilities to fulfil their caring roles. This was reflected not just in the actions of family and friends, or among professionals working in social care, but also in the public and private sectors more broadly. Carers with learning disabilities talked of having their role as carer ignored or dismissed as their own personal problem by employers and by leisure and health professionals. Several participants talked about having to give up paid work or being unable to complete college courses in order to care for their loved ones and discussed how difficult it had been to have their caring roles recognised and receive support to continue to pursue their own lives as well as provide care. Two of the carers had tried to gain support from their employers, asking for flexible working times. One reported a dismissive response from the manager who 'said he didn't want to know my problems'. The other person had initially had a more positive response but the promised offer of assistance had not been forthcoming and the person had ultimately had to resign. Other participants talked about health and social care professionals not including them in discussions and decision making, even though they were the main care giver. Examples included hospitals not talking to the person with learning disability about their parents' illness and care needs, insisting on talking to a sibling instead, or paid support workers talking in hushed tones with siblings when the care giver left the room. In this way the carers with learning disabilities demonstrated the importance of a collective responsibility for recognising the need for care in order to successfully support caring relationships.

Responsibility: caring for

Tronto suggests that responsibility is not something solely located with the individual, but something that exists in the 'relationships among people' (2013, p 50). It is not therefore about the expression of paternalistic power, within which we might talk of one person taking responsibility for another and therefore taking power away from them. Robinson (1999, p 25) discusses the notion of respect joined with care – a useful way of conceptualising responsibility in this context. Responsibility is about the act of caring for another, but it derives from attentiveness to their position and is therefore about delivering care with respect. For people with learning disabilities who are carers this was expressed both in their recognition of the skills and needs of those with whom they were in a caring relationship and also in the ways that they discussed the relationship and their roles within it. People talked about shared tasks, about the things that they did and also the things that the person they cared for did in ways that were explicitly representative of mutual interdependence. Similarly, when they discussed being a carer this was often framed in a way that showed respect for the feelings of their loved one. One person who cared for his mother said 'Caring isn't a word I'd use, I just help her out. You're not to be my carer she said, she wants to do things her way'; while another woman suggested 'When it's your mum and dad you don't think of it as caring, you are just proud to do it, I mean after everything they have done for me.' Responsibility as considered in care ethics is not about obligation. While the carers we talked to here did sometimes talk about doing the right thing and returning the care they had been shown, as indicated above, the emphasis was on reciprocal and mutual care relationships. As such, responsibility here was expressed through a relational mutuality that acknowledges interdependence and engenders self-esteem, mutual respect, trust and responsibility (Robinson, 1999, p 48). One of the difficulties in discussing responsibility in the context of care ethics is considering where the responsibility lies, which can be an ambiguous process (Tronto, 2013, p 51). While people with learning disabilities may be seen to be expressing relational mutuality by caring for those that have and do care for them, they also experience barriers in exercising this responsibility. Everyone who took part in the Fulfilling Potential consultation noted that caring was an important responsibility suggesting that being a carer *'makes you a good person, more responsible'*. However, as indicated above, many also noted that it was a role that was not recognised by professionals or other family members and this made it more difficult for them to care for their loved ones. One explicit example of this came from a woman who lived in a relationship of mutual care with her mother but within which only her mother received a carer's allowance. Her mother had been identified as the main carer for many years and, despite the fact that she now needed support with shopping, cooking and bathing, she was still seen as the care giver in the relationship. This mutual care is something that policy fails to recognise, requiring as it does a bifurcation of the roles of care receiver and care giver, the presumption being that the care receiver is so dependent that they could not possibly also provide care. The lack of recognition was also reflected in the fact that many people found it hard to recognise themselves as carers and hadn't realised that they had significant caring roles until someone pointed it out to them. The very language of being a carer was not one that was available to people with learning disabilities. Previous research has demonstrated that many carers' organisations either do not recognise or do not understand the particular needs of carers who have learning disabilities (Holman et al, 2009). Tronto notes that the person or group who are assigned responsibility also need 'sufficient power to carry out the assignment' (2013, p 51). For people with learning difficulties their own marginalisation and positioning can make this difficult. They report experiences in which either they are seen as incapable of exercising such responsibility or, as indicated above, other people involved in the matrices of care – often professionals – take steps to 'protect' them from the responsibility.

People with learning disabilities who are carers also recognise the importance in their lives of others who demonstrate the ability to respond to them in a way that enhances the care relationship and provides support:

> "The people at my church let me make tea and coffee every Sunday and they are very kind and they talk to me and one of them takes Mum and I to [the] Garden Centre."

> "I was referred to a youth club for young adults with autism for two hours each week. That made all the difference. I'm too old now for the club but they are talking to me about being a volunteer."

What these examples illustrate is the importance of networked care and having opportunities to enact reciprocity both within and beyond the dyadic care relationship. It was important both to be able to demonstrate responsibility and also to have others show responsibility in caring for them in order to sustain the networks of care.

Competence: care giving

Competence may be seen as having the ability to care not just physically, by going through the motions of tending to someone, but in a way that is embedded in relational mutuality. To simply tend to an issue without embedding that response in care can be seen as an act of 'bad faith' (Tronto, 1993, p 133). In this way competence needs to be considered alongside the notions of attentiveness and responsibility. As noted above, people with learning disabilities who are carers demonstrated competence by attending to the needs of the person they were caring for and using their skills to assist where and when help was needed. The participants talked about being involved in wide range of physical tasks that included reading letters, shopping, cooking, paying bills, assisting with personal care, calling for help when someone had a fall and helping with medication. In so doing they also demonstrated continued attentiveness, and amended the care they gave according to changing needs. This was summarised by one son who said:

"Over time I do more odd jobs for my mum because her arthritis got so bad. I had to do it as she used to drop things on the floor."

Carers with a learning disability also demonstrated their competence by recognising the importance of updating their skills and having appropriate support; so they identified the need for training and accessible information so that they would know what support was available and from where. While the carers we spoke to demonstrated competence in their caring roles they also recognised the need for support in these roles and, even more significantly, they recognised the way that the views of others towards them could hamper them in their caring roles. Having their competence acknowledged was important to people with learning disabilities who were carers, not only in order to get appropriate support, but also because they recognised that they were viewed differently when they had a valued role in society such as being a carer or working. Those who participated in the consultation thought that there needed to be more awareness, particularly within public services providing health and social care, that people with learning disabilities can be carers (Baker et al, 2012). When discussing these points they referred to the need for professionals to receive training so that they could work more effectively in supporting carers who have a learning disability. In this way they recognised that their own competence as carers was influenced by the competence of others.

Responsiveness: care receiving

Within care ethics responsiveness focuses our gaze onto the care receiver as we consider their response to care. For those who were caring for parents, grandparents and siblings, the 'care receiver' had, throughout much of their lives, been recognised by service providers and other family members as the care giver. In mutual caring roles, where the person with a learning disability had increasingly taken on a caring role, tensions were sometimes apparent. People with learning disabilities who were carers sometimes found it difficult to exercise their independence. One man who had spent some years caring for his mother noted that he wasn't allowed to go out much because his mother and the paid carers didn't want him to, often wanting him to stay in the house even at times when they were there to provide respite. Another male carer agreed, saying:

"I would like to go out a bit more. I have just got a girlfriend and haven't told Mum about it in case she doesn't want me to see her. Mum is scared about being on her own for too long."

For some of the care receivers this related to fears of being left, while in others it reflected the protective role that the care receiver had been used to taking in the relationship. In some instances this played out in more controlling and disempowering ways, for example one person who did receive a carer's allowance said that their mother "kept saying you can't go out you are paid to stay with me all the time". Engster argues that

> Responsiveness means engaging in some form of dialogue with others in order to discern the precise nature of their needs, and monitoring their responses to our care (whether verbal or nonverbal) to make sure they are receiving what they need. (Engster, 2005, p 54)

When considering this in terms of relationships of mutual care the negotiation of these needs becomes increasingly complex and, it could be argued, is representative of an important expression of relational morality. People with learning disabilities who are carers were seen to do this by holding in balance their own needs alongside those of the people they were caring for, and for many this extended beyond the immediate care receiver to others involved in networks of care through a process of liaison and negotiation. So people talked about having to liaise with professional service providers to ensure that direct payments worked smoothly, monitoring the care provided by paid support staff to ensure that they were doing their job effectively and raising concerns if this was not the case, and keeping other members of the family informed about key issues. In so doing it is also apparent that the carers who have learning disabilities draw on previous experience and transferrable skills. In this way they are demonstrating through their actions the interconnectedness of these different aspects of care ethics, demonstrating their competence as carers while acting responsibly to ensure that the situation is responsive to on-going and changing needs.

For Tronto, responsiveness also requires that we remain alert 'to the possibilities for abuse that arise with vulnerability' (1993, p 135). This is particularly important when considering the position of people with learning disabilities who are carers, where assumptions about their vulnerability and capacity can lead to a lack of recognition and could possibly be used as a justification for them not be accorded rights as care givers. The lack of recognition makes people with learning disabilities who are carers particularly vulnerable to a lack of care as carers and is, I would argue, representative of a failure to care on the part of professionals. Sometimes the person being cared for wants/needs the care giver to do something that they may find uncomfortable. For example, one man said: "I would like it if Mum let the carer lady shower her on a Monday, then I wouldn't have to do it." If a care relationship is to be responsive, then the subjective experience and needs of both the care giver and the care receiver need to be acknowledged. Whereas in many relationships of care the care giver is usually deemed to hold the power, this is not the case for people with learning difficulties who are carers. Throughout their lives they have been perceived as vulnerable and dependent and this therefore makes it more difficult for them to be recognised as carers or to stand up for their rights. These traditional roles and assumptions can obscure transitions in family life and the development of mutual and nested caring relationships.

Conclusions: caring morality, reciprocity and mutual care

Gilligan (1993) argues that moral maturity is not purely about the application of abstract and objective thought. In discussing their experiences of their roles as carers, people with learning disabilities demonstrate a moral maturity in their care. They engage with a range of others in this relationship, weighing and assessing the right thing to do. In developing this moral maturity they draw on their own experiences of care, and of being cared for, in order to understand and attend to the needs and positions of those they then come to care for, as well as their own needs as carers. Deliberating with care in difficult and sometimes highly affective situations is in many ways a much more complex skill than objective thought.

Care is often reduced to a personal, private activity and one that does not involve a high level of skills – and this is reflected in the low levels of pay and recognition that care work attracts. Care is also often portrayed as a vocation, an activity that involves self-sacrifice. Through their experiences as care givers the carers with learning disabilities who took part in this consultation came to understand care as a far more complex activity that was part of a web of reciprocity and mutuality that involved not just self-sacrifice but also the importance of reciprocity and self-care – they experienced at first hand what Tronto talks of when she suggests that care is a species activity that enables us to maintain our world as a world that 'includes our bodies, ourselves, and our environment, all of which we seek to interweave in a complex, life-sustaining web' (Tronto, 1993, p 103).

While the failure to be attentive may be a moral failing (Tronto, 1993), in the context of mutual and nested relationships of care it becomes necessary to explore where the moral failing lies. People with learning disabilities who are carers experience barriers to the fulfilment of their caring roles, there is a lack of attentiveness, an absence of care, that makes it difficult for them to fulfil their caring roles and also impacts on those they are caring for. The moral failure here is not that of the carer who has a learning disability, or of the person being cared for. It lies with the policy makers who constrain our views of the care relationship into narrow, dyadic notions that distinguish the carer and the cared for; and with workers who are ignorant of the impact of changing relationships of care, who do not see – and are therefore unable to support – the carer who has a learning disability.

This chapter has shown the importance of reciprocity and mutuality in relationships of care and has explored the way that people with learning disabilities who are carers demonstrate the different aspects of care ethics in their roles. These moral elements of care are not only intertwined (Tronto, 1993, p 136), with each relating to the other: they may also be seen to connect to the activities of all of those involved in the relationship of care. Considering this in relation to mutual and nested relationships of care suggests the need to broaden our understanding of attentiveness so that it understands the needs of all of those in the care relationship from their subjective positions. Doing so will provide a more nuanced understanding of the power and positionality involved in relationships of care and so be more likely to recognise and provide spaces for expressions of responsibility, to support the development of competence and therefore enable responsiveness within the complex reality of changing and nested relationships of care.

Acknowledgement

The research that influenced the ideas in this chapter was conducted by the author in conjunction with Lucy Virgo, Kelley Johnson and Cath Baker, along with members of the Carers with Learning Disabilities Network. Thanks go to the members of the network and all of the people who participated in the consultation for agreeing to share their experiences of care.

FOURTEEN

People with intellectual disabilities (visually) reimagine care

Ann Fudge Schormans

Introduction

Care is typically understood as both a value and a practice. The practice of care – who is cared for, how and by whom – typically reflects societal values and the (de)valuation of particular groups of people. As a practice, care 'invokes different experiences, different meanings, different contexts and multiple relations of power, of which a political argument around care needs to take account' (Williams, 2001, p 468).

Highlighting the perspective of the disabled care receiver, disability scholars have challenged accepted notions of care and care practices for disabled people. As articulated elsewhere in this collection (Chapter One), for many in the disabled people's movement the word 'care' has become synonymous with the pathologisation and medicalisation of impairment and disability (Power, 2010), with exclusion, disempowerment and loss of rights: an oppressive practice to be actively resisted (Hughes, McKie, Hopkins and Watson, 2005).

Visual media representations of disability are similarly understood as pathologising and reductive (Elks, 2005). This matters because, despite their nature as socially constructed and functional, visual representations are typically received uncritically, regarded as 'truth'. As such, they influence the meanings and value we ascribe to others (Derrida, 2001) and how we treat these 'others' as a consequence. Relying on dysfunctional and dehumanising stereotypes, they reflect and shape cultural assumptions about disability, vulnerability, dependence and care (Garland-Thomson, 2001): for example, people with impairment as eternal children, helpless, unable and burden (Hevey, 1997). As a practice of power, such images are sites of oppression, of un-care (Butler, 2004).

Tying together and complicating these two concerns – care and visual representation of disability – is the argument that while the larger disability community (particularly people with physical or sensory disability) rejects dominant notions of care that paint disabled people as unable and needy in favour of self-directed support (Kröger, 2009), this same community has seldom attended to the situations or perspectives of people labelled with intellectual disabilities (ID). The emphasis on agency over care has meant that the need for (sometimes lifelong) support and dependence on others of some persons with ID – especially those who may find it more difficult to do for themselves or to direct their own care – and our understanding of how care is defined, experienced and practised by persons with ID have not been adequately theorised: an unintended consequence may be perpetuation of the devaluation of people with ID (Kittay, 2001b; Yong, 2007). This may also obscure alternative understandings of what care might be, the forms it might take, how and by whom it might be provided, and how it might be experienced differently. Further, while (and, in part, because) public visual representations typically construct people with ID as unable and dependent, this group has been denied the opportunity to engage in these debates – to speak to disabling visual constructions and articulate their own understandings of and need for care (Fudge Schormans and Chambon, 2012).

Engaging with a political ethic of care and disability studies critique of care, this chapter will share some of the work done by a group of adults with ID with public photographic representations of the care of people so labelled. The work revealed many considerations of their experiences and understandings of ID and care *and* of visual representations *as* care. Included are questions of vulnerability, protection, love, touch and their unfortunate converse. Triggered by their engagement with the images and their critique of the images as sites of care or oppression, the complexity and primacy of notions of care and care practices to people with ID was revealed as an on-going tension in group members' lives and is expressed in their work with the images.

The 'What's wrong with this picture?' project

The work under discussion emerged from a study that made use of inclusive research ideologies and arts-informed methodologies to explore the ways public photographic images represent persons with ID, influencing cultural understandings of who they are and might be, what they need and how they should be treated. Attending to the on-going marginalisation of people with ID in research about them, the project was concerned with learning how people with ID themselves would see and respond to these cultural representations and means of knowing; and how they might use photography to disrupt these disabling representations and understandings.

Four people self-identifying as having ID joined me in this project – Sam, Bob, Donna and Robin (note, in publications and presentations of their work, they insist on use of their first names). They worked individually and collectively with their selection of 11 public photographic images of people with ID (drawn from newspapers, advertising, service organisation materials, photographic art and social documentary sources). They first engaged in critical discussions about the images, speaking to their immediate reactions, the messages about ID that they believed the images conveyed, how they felt non-disabled others might interpret and respond to the images, and the potential consequences to their own lives and those of others with ID. A digital media specialist used the computer software program Photoshop to help the group to transform these images as a means to visually realise their critique. He also took new photographs that they directed and approved. The final step of the project was a series of art gallery-styled exhibits curated by group members and presented to different audiences. In these exhibits the group's counter-images were strategically paired with the originals: a political move that unsettled accepted notions of people labelled ID, their understanding of the world and their position in it, and their ability to articulate such in creative and powerful ways (for further details on the project's structure and audience responses, see Fudge Schormans, 2011 and 2015 and Fudge Schormans and Chambon, 2012).

Important here is that through their work with these images they articulated a complexity of meaning and experience of care, the necessity and meaningfulness of particular types of care and how, for them, care might be reimagined otherwise. It is not possible in this chapter to do justice to the depth or scope of their work, but let me share their work with one photographic image – of a 14 year-old-girl and a care giver – and the counter-images they created in response. Regrettably, I am not able to reproduce the image here. While a number of the photographers and/or copyright holders of the images used in this project were wonderfully supportive of (and interested in) the group's use of their images, others were less so. For example, one simply did not answer repeated e-mails seeking permission for use of the image (the e-mail address had been confirmed); another withdrew permission to reproduce her/his image upon viewing the group's transformation(s) and hearing their critique of it; and from a third I received only a very short and (what I interpreted to be) terse refusal. My e-mail request to discuss this was not answered.

As a practice of power, it is necessary to consider what these refusals might mean. These responses raise additional questions: about ableist perceptions of people with ID and about care. As already noted, public visual representations often reveal dominant cultural ideas about the disabled 'other'. In seeming to reflect and (once again) reproduce long-standing assumptions as to the (in)ability of many people with ID to have both opinions on how they have been represented and the ability and desire to share such with others (Fudge Schormans and Chambon, 2012), and to deny them their right to do so, arguably, these refusals work to silence and disempower people with ID. As such, they signal both a lack of care and yet another example of subjugation. Disallowing the reproduction and broader distribution of the group's work with the images, complicating their ability to engage in on-going debates about the visual representation of ID and people so labelled, perpetuates oppressive imagery as a site of un-care. But if one does not believe people with ID to be capable of critique, why suppress their counter-images? I cannot help but wonder whether the potential power and value of the critique was recognised and understood to be somehow threatening. In the immediacy of this chapter, however, these copyright restrictions mean that I must rely on textual descriptions of the original image and the group's counter-images. In these descriptions I have attempted both to do justice to the group's work with the images and to be as respectful of the girl and her carer as possible.

Vulnerability, dependency and the need for care

This colour image, taken from a Canadian newspaper, is set in a clinical setting – a small, dark room with pale grey walls and carpet, white draperies and no visible wall decorations. The light from a lamp with a white shade that sits atop a small bedside table (also holding a book) shines down onto the face of 14-year-old girl sitting in the arms of her carer. Close behind these two figures, in the corner of the room, underneath the window, is a single bed. It is covered with a white mattress sheet but no blankets, pillow or bedspread: the bottom mattress (dark blue, with diagonal white stripes and white edging) and a mechanism to lift and lower the bed can be clearly seen. Resting against the plain dark headboard are a foam neck support and a yellow-striped stuffed toy.

The left half of the image is consumed by a large black wheelchair – exceeding the image's frame (not all of the chair is captured within the photograph) exaggerates its size. The wheelchair has a dark blue cover on the seat, back and side rests (which appear customised to support the girl's body), support straps are visible, as is an unidentifiable piece of equipment propped in the seat. Its positioning obstructs much of the bed. Somewhat diminished by the wheelchair and the girl she is holding, the figure of the carer (who we learn from the accompanying article is the girl's foster mother) is sitting in a dark-coloured, armless chair positioned perpendicular to the bed and to the right of the wheelchair. Blond, curly-haired, she wears glasses and, around her neck, a pendant that lies atop a bright red sweatshirt. She wears a large watch on her right wrist, blue jeans and white socks (and what appears to be a pink slipper is lying on the floor beside her left foot) and she is holding the girl on her lap, arms wrapped around the girl's waist, hands clasped together. She faces the girl so that we see only her profile. Her eyes focused on the girl's face, she is smiling.

The girl is wearing bright blue pants – seemingly too long, as they wrinkle, bunch and gather around her slender legs; the bottoms are tucked into dark blue, down-filled slipper-boots. She also wears a long-sleeved white shirt. Her slight body – seemingly much longer than that of the carer – is sprawled across the woman's lap. With legs bent at the knees and falling to the right, feet resting on the floor, her lower half seems to rest largely on the woman's right thigh. Her upper body is arched back at the waist such that it lies perpendicular to the floor. Both arms – bent at the elbows – drop backwards away from her body, her long fingers are curled; her head similarly appears to be falling backwards and looks almost as if it has come to rest atop the night table behind her. The girl's pale face is turned towards the ceiling, her dark hair falling away from her face. Eyes shut, mouth slightly open – a semi-circle of light from the bedside table lamp shines upon and frames her face, thus making it the brightest spot of the image.

> Ann: OK, alright, what do you think, Donna? What do you think this picture is about?
>
> Donna: It's about, like, that she has a disability, (pause) this just reminds me that she can't walk and she can't feed herself …
>
> Sam: Yeah, that's exactly what I was going to say!
>
> Donna: … and she can't even go to the washroom herself, so … and she can't wash herself…. Yeah, she needs *a lot* of help!

Looking at this image, the group members were immediately drawn to the girl's body. They remarked often upon its positioning, its shape and size. Believing non-disabled viewers would regard the girl as 'scary' and not quite human (as they themselves report being regarded), they questioned the decision to photograph her in this way. They noted how her long body and flailing limbs – exaggerated by the camera – are represented as seeming to overwhelm the care giver tightly holding her, emphasising vulnerability and inability (that of the girl *and* the care giver) and burden. They were angered at how this excessively staged representation both makes plain and exaggerates her impairment.

The wheelchair similarly arrested their attention. Consuming half of the image, it operates as visual shorthand to further define the girl and, in emphasising what she cannot do, conveys the 'facts' of her impairment and dependence; she needs others to do *for* her. Alert to the constructed nature of the image, they voiced their belief that the mere presence of a wheelchair in a photograph tells viewers the person is disabled; there is 'something wrong'. Abetted by the hospital bed and other pieces of equipment in the image, they argued that this is what the photographer intended it to do. This is not a personal photograph of this girl, one that tells us about who she is as a person or her life outside of this room and this moment. Instead, it has been framed to tell us *only* what she cannot do and, in so doing, to inform viewers what others must do for her. Yet, they themselves understood her to be vulnerable and in need of care: 'because the person just can't function like [the non-disabled] you can, like normal, can't function as normally as you can, she has to be in a wheelchair and cared for all the time'. For the group, the girl's dependence was largely unquestioned: her impairment is 'real' and it poses barriers – she cannot, in any great measure, do for herself or direct others towards the provision of that which she must have. Impairment, vulnerability, dependency and the need for care are, in this case, co-extensive.

Listening to these conversations, I wondered whether the group's thoughts were indicative of their inculcation into pathologising discourses that, in valorising autonomy and independence while simultaneously stigmatising vulnerability and dependency, serve to devalue people with impairments. Had they fallen prey to the disabling production of people with ID in public photographic representations? Their responses to the image made clear that they recognised it as one of constructed excess, yet, for the group, the girl's dependence *is* a taken-for-granted 'truth', and is understood to be different from that of other disabled people who can, for instance, direct their own support needs. Throughout the project, they identified with the subjects of the images to the extent that they too have intellectual and other impairments that similarly create 'problems' for them. They too sometimes require care and support. They also know other people with ID who have physical impairments and support needs such as this girl has. With an empathy seemingly born of this shared identification as a person with ID, they did not, however, construe this dependence negatively.

> Robin: That's how [the person in the image] was born, like that.
> Bob: Some people are like that.
> Donna: I don't think there's [anything] wrong with anybody who has a disability, I don't find – you're born like that, that's the way life is. God made you like that. You can't do anything about it.

For the group members, the girl's need for care is unremarkable: what is critical is what this need for care can lead to.

Seeing un-care

What the group members came to see in this image was un-care. Other images they worked with evoked similar reactions and were similarly understood to represent and reproduce the devaluation and experiences of un-care that they themselves – along with so many people with ID – endure. The disabled subjects of these photographs were regarded as being vulnerable, in need of but not receiving care; neither from those charged with their actual care, nor from these visual representations. Vulnerability was understood to leave one open and susceptible to hurt and for this girl (and people with ID in other images) the group's concern over her need for care was matched, if not exceeded, by their worries that the care she required was not being provided, was inadequate or, worse, might actually be harming her. For example, they believed the position of her body (for example, her arched back) was uncomfortable and painful. She seems at risk of banging her head on the table behind her – when Robin and Sam first viewed this photograph, they believed she had done this and had been killed as a result. The diminutive care giver grasping her so awkwardly seems unable to keep her from falling and, thus, from harm.

The more the group members looked, the more 'bad care' they saw. They questioned whether the girl's impairment was not, at least in part, an effect of this un-care. The care giver seems unable to support the girl. The setting is cold, unwelcoming and medicalised. They wondered why the care giver is smiling – does she believe that the care she is providing (or the image itself) is OK? That this is how people with ID should be treated? That they deserve no better? Struggling with the possibility that non-disabled others would regard people with ID as so undeserving and thus see this care and the image as acceptable, they found the image 'hard to look at' and wanted not to see it. It was painful to view because they looked upon the girl not as an object, nor even as the subject of this photograph, but as a real person who, like themselves, had been identified as having an ID. Engaging not only with the image but also with the 'real' person within it, they repeatedly expressed their desire to 'meet and talk to the girl', to give her 'support and a hug'. Theirs is a caring gaze; they are concerned about her and outraged that others are not similarly caring.

The group searched for alternative and more acceptable ways of imaging the girl's need for care. Over the course of several conversations, a consensus emerged that just as the girl's life is more complex than this image suggests, so too are the meanings of care and notions of how it should be provided.

Picturing care differently

You have to tell the 'right' story

In their first re-telling and re-imagining of the girl's story, a re-telling that makes plain one meaning of care this image provokes for them, they chose (in some ways reminiscent of the photographer of the original image) to concentrate upon the girl's physical vulnerability, her dependence and need for support. Their first act was to remove the girl and carer from the clinical setting of the original. A plain but bright white background denounces the prescriptive scene they read in the original: the clinical environment is no longer the necessary (and thus best or only) space for people with impairment; instead they make possible a multitude of spaces for her by identifying the setting with the label 'MY OWN ACCESSIBLE APARTMENT', placed in the bottom left of the image. Photoshop was used to cut the figures of the carer (still in the chair) and the girl (still in her arms) from the original; however, Photoshop was further used to alter the girl's posture, to position her sitting upright in the carer's lap. The figures were then placed in the centre of the transformed image (occupying more of the right side than of the left). The label 'love' was placed above the woman's hands. Disrupting the clinical scene of the original even further, behind and to the right of the carer and girl is a decorative wooden door – of the type one would expect to see in a home or apartment. The label 'funding' has been placed on the door; the universal symbol of accessibility has been placed beside it (on the right).

Behind the figures, and now clearly visible, is a hospital bed – a more specialised and well-equipped bed than that in the original. This one has safety bars, is in a raised position, and has a motorised mattress and additional pad (both to facilitate comfort) lying atop it. The label 'special equipment' has been placed on the bed. Behind and left of the bed is a smaller wheelchair (not the original, as this proved too difficult to Photoshop out of the original image) and, while it does not have an individualised seating form, it is intended to indicate that the wheelchair is neither the most important nor singularly defining feature of either the room or the girl. A blonde-haired woman wearing a white shirt (which may or may not be a nursing uniform) and holding her hands together stands behind the wheelchair with her body angled towards the girl and carer, her smiling face turned towards the viewer. Beside her is the label 'people to support me'.

Citing the insufficiency of the original image, and drawing upon their personal experience as developmental service users and self-advocates, the group elected to provide concrete information about the types of support the girl requires and to construct their transformation around this. Mixing both clinical and non-clinical elements, they included information about where she should live and how accessible the place should be; the availability of support persons; necessary and top-quality equipment; and financial support. Limiting the space taken up by the wheelchair facilitated this. They wanted the viewer to know more about what (they believed) her daily life is/could be like and what is required to make that life 'good'. They labelled these things in their transformation, so as to emphasise and make plain what 'good care' requires.

I was curious about this seemingly mechanistic, service-based rendering that, in losing the girl amid the itemised supports, seemed to fly in the face of their critique of the image. I asked for explanations and was told that the inclusion of more information would enable viewers to learn about the girl's life and what she needs. Challenging the devaluation of the need for care that they saw in the original, they interrupted the emphasis in the original image on the girl's body by changing her posture, sitting her upright. They know she can sit upright – the wheelchair tells them this. They stated that what was required was more detail as to the supports that should be in place: 'How is the picture going to actually tell the story if you don't actually see everything that's in the picture properly?' They proffered this as the means by which to educate non-disabled people in a way that cares for people with ID.

While the group continued to highlight the girl's dependence, they simultaneously attributed to her agency, thus further troubling the original image. Their changes were rooted in what they believe to be the girl's preferences – 'she would/wouldn't want …' – thus foregrounding the girl over the supports and insisting that her choices be honoured. I am not sure if they believed she could direct her own supports or if, in acknowledging her impairments, they were speaking not so much *for* her as from their shared position as people with ID – from a knowing, an attentiveness, rooted in this position, with her or even *as* her. Either way, they made the girl present, and I began to see how their transformation reflected their caring. By sitting her upright they made it easier for the care giver to hold her, as well as correct the physical hurt they presumed to be done to the girl through the awkward positioning of her body. She also looks less 'scary' or 'strange', thus humanising her by countering the dysfunctional representation of her body in the original image. The transformed image is a more care-full one that no longer harms her. More than this, it makes room – and a more suitable room/space – for her, for her differences, thus inviting new understandings. In the minds of the group, it will lead to better care. Now that the viewer can see and thus know what people living with her type of impairment need and have the right to receive, they will be provoked to action and will 'try to do something about it'. By telling the 'right' story the group create an opening to effect change, hoping that, with knowledge, people will do the 'right thing'.

Seeing care, love, and protection

Audible in much of the group's discussion of the original image was the notion that something good was contained within. It was Sam who noted that while the care giver's hold on the girl is precarious, it might also be understood as a 'hug': 'the girl is sitting on the care giver's lap for a little close company', for 'loving or caring'. The care giver's smile was reinterpreted as an expression of love. And in the first transformation, group members identified 'love' as one of the things the girl needs. Love was understood as a form of care and the word itself was deliberately placed near the care giver's hands wrapped around the girl; it was set upon her heart.

Returning to this in later conversations, the group distinguished between 'caring for' and 'caring about', arguing that the former is dependent upon the latter. If people (care givers, photographers, non-disabled people) 'really cared' about people with ID, then people with ID would receive better care and these types of representations would cease to exist. From this emerged a second interpretation and visual representation of care. Moving beyond what is practically required in the provision of 'care for' people with ID, this second transformation exemplified the group's affective concern with 'caring about': with care as love and loving care.

In the group's discussions, protection became entangled with love for this girl and for the subjects of other images whom they similarly regarded as being in real danger. The girl being unable to care for herself, her well-being, her very life depends upon others meeting her needs – on her being kept safe. The girl concerned them and they professed caring about her. Focusing on the loving and protective relationship captured by the care giver's arms wrapped around the girl, representing this type of holding became paramount. This is the love and protection they want the girl *and themselves* to receive, for they too have been hurt by care and expect to be hurt again. They shared all-too-common experiences of having been placed in positions of enforced dependence on service providers and family members; of feeling powerless yet aware of the risks entailed in resistance (see Fudge Schormans, 2014); of hurtful service-based relationships with 'paid' staff who they felt did not care about them; and of feeling unloved and rejected. They told me that in this world there are people who are wanted, and those who are not. The girl in the image – like them – falls into the latter category. Their words point to another side of un-care – there is also wanting; wanting to be someone who is wanted. They wished to modify the image to make obvious that the holding, the relationship, is a caring *and* a safe one; to focus 'on the grip, like make sure it's tight'. They told me that if someone '*really* loved her' they would hold the girl properly and keep her safe. With love comes an un-refusable responsibility to protect against harm. With love, comes good care.

The group's second transformation, then, would tell a different story. They chose not to include the wheelchair, bed or medical equipment – the markers of impairment and (service) dependence dominating the scene in the original and first transformed images. They chose, instead, to highlight or 'make bigger' the touch, the loving relationship; to make plain that 'care' is much more than attending only to physical support needs. Rejecting again the less pleasurable clinical scene of the original, they used Photoshop to place the girl and care giver in a 'nicer place', 'a park', where they could 'sit on a bench' and 'enjoy the day' and each other's company. By adhering more to the style of portraiture, the modified (upright) figure of the girl and the carer lovingly embracing her are made the central focus of this transformed image. Placed against a background of trees and bright blue sky, this time we see these figures not in their entirety, but only to the level of the upper thighs. The label 'love' (indeed, all labels) has been removed. Barely visible through the trees are high-rise buildings and a road being travelled by a few cars, indicating that the park is in a city of some size.

Discussion

Politicising public photographic images of (un)care

It is generally understood that visual images have the power to influence our perceptions of 'same' and 'different' (Derrida, 2001) and to 'other' particular groups of people (Butler, 2004). Created primarily by non-disabled others, the exercise of power over disabled people evident in public photographic imagery has resulted in much harm (Garland-Thomson, 2001). In unity with the disabled people's movement, the group's critique of the photograph of the girl reveals that they are alert to how the vulnerability and dependency of people with ID are made to be 'hypervisible' (Kittay, 2001b, p 570), and the domination and oppression accruing as a result. Linking this specifically to care, what people do, how they do (not) provide care, is tangled up with the meanings ascribed to receivers of care (Barnes and Brannelly, 2008). That the images are deliberately staged, that people with ID are purposefully constructed in such dehumanising ways, led the group to regard these photographs as images of the specific suffering of people with ID, images expressing 'the individual pain' that is their experience of devaluation (Green, Mann and Story, 2006, p 177). The hurtful treatment of people with ID cannot be attributed to a few 'bad people': reflecting their belief that most non-disabled people 'just don't care' about people with ID, the group understood these images as a collective practice of un-care.

The group struggled with how the images 'don't tell the truth about people with ID'. This they believed dangerous for a number of reasons. First, by failing to more accurately reveal who people with ID are, the complexity of their lives and what they both need and have a right to receive, people's needs cannot be met. Second, because there are so few alternative visual representations of people with ID existing images effect a capture of labelled people, fostering the belief that they are all the same and should be treated the same way. More egregiously, they reinforce notions that the 'bad care' evident in the images is somehow acceptable, and even deserved.

The group also came to realise that, when used by and in the service of people with ID, visual imagery can begin to disrupt the relationship between 'care, domination, and representation' (Green et al, 2006, p 177). Important here is how their shared label of ID enables a particular type of attentiveness to the disabled subjects of the images: they recognise these subjects (they *are* these subjects), they feel – and reject – the (un) care being inflicted, they want/demand better. Believing themselves responsible to the girl in the image, group members feel called to 'a posture of care' (p 178). Their transformations are intended not only as political and ethical *critique* of care and care practices, but also as a political and ethical *practice* of care; an expression of attentiveness, responsiveness and responsibility (Barnes and Brannelly, 2008), of their own caring for and about the disabled subjects in the images.

Photographic representation as an ethical and political practice of care

The two transformations of the image of the girl, in picturing care differently, call into question accepted notions of care for people with ID. Aligning with the disabled people's movement and a political ethic of care, the first asserts the girl's right of access to needed supports and to the exercise of agency over provision of these supports, challenging assumptions that one cannot be both in need of care and capable of agency and empowerment (Kröger, 2009). The second emphasises that people with ID have the right, and should expect to receive, care that is not hurtful, that takes place outside of institutionalised/medicalised contexts and supports a life well lived and of one's own choosing. Both transformations demonstrate that the girl – irrespective of her dependence on others for care – is valued: by the woman holding her, and by the group members.

The group's affective and care-full (Fudge Schormans, 2011) responses to the image – their recognition of and attentiveness to the *real* person in the image and the multiplicity of what she needs/ wants – reflects their position as one not of gazing at but of caring for and about the girl. The emotional and relational contexts of care are foundational to the practice of 'good care'. Unintentionally engaging with debates as to the role of emotional attachment in care (Barnes and Brannelly, 2008; Kröger, 2009), they appear to share Thomas's belief that 'our embodied selves also require ongoing emotional sustenance – to receive and to give personal appreciation, affection and love – if we are to be "fully human"' (Thomas, 2007, p 87) and to believe that this should take place in care relationships.

This attentiveness necessitates the group members assumption of responsibility both to and for the girl, a sense of responsibility extending to the disabled subjects of other images, themselves and all people with ID. Aware of the heterogeneity of persons labelled ID, they spoke frequently of how their individual needs for 'support', 'help', 'assistance' – for care – differed from each other's and from those of the subjects of the images. Recognising dependency as 'an irrevocable and general fact of existence' (Green et al, 2006, p 180), as rooted in the vulnerability of the body, they understand too that '[a]ll of us are vulnerable, then, but certainly not equally vulnerable' (Green et al, 2006, p 181). Their own care needs were not the same as those of the girl in the image, whom they understood to have more complex impairments, to be more vulnerable and dependent. However, this was no reason to distance themselves from her, as some within the disability movement are accused of doing (O'Hara, 2008). To the contrary, this led group members to regard themselves as being responsible to act (Barnes and Brannelly, 2008), to rectify the un-care perpetrated in and through the image.

Group members understood that in this instance they (unlike the girl) had the power to change the image and thus effect a re-imaging and reimagining of care for the girl. Responsive to her vulnerability, they believed themselves similarly responsive to her preferences/choices/desires for care. The artificiality of the circumstances of their enactment of responsiveness and responsibility arguably invites challenge. The care provided through their transformations was done from their suppositions as to what the girl would want, which was, without doubt, largely informed by their own position/experience as people with ID – as service users, care receivers and self-advocates. Yet this position, and their caring about the girl, might begin to work towards facilitating the type of attentiveness and responsiveness to another that is necessary to understanding what that other person requires (Barnes and Brannelly, 2008; O'Hara, 2008).

Conclusion

Both the disabled people's movement and those engaging with a political ethic of care demand that we pay attention to our understanding of care and care practices for disabled people, that we picture care differently and do so from the experiential knowledge of care receivers (Kröger, 2009). Like the disabled people's movement, the group struggled with accepted notions of care and the devaluation of people with ID, understood to be dependent, that they saw in the images and had personal experience of. For them, 'care' often 'hurts', physically *and* emotionally. They saw many of the people in the images as uncared for, unloved, isolated – in group homes, segregated classes, institutions, abandoned in and to the image – and made plain the divide between the person with ID and the non-disabled, un-caring carer. But, they did not embrace the movement's *exclusive* focus on self-directed support, on liberal notions of autonomy that continue to devalue the need for care (Barnes, 2011). While the vulnerability and dependency of people with ID have been a 'foundation for domination' and thus something to be fought against, they are also a fact of all our lives as human beings and 'the source of the ethical call to care' (Green et al, 2006, p 191). Believing themselves called to care, the group enacted their own practice of care through visually re-imaging and reimagining care. By using their power 'in a positive and creative manner' (Barnes and Brannelly, 2008, p 386), their transformations of the image of the girl begin to challenge the limited and reductive ideas of how care could/should be provided to people with ID that they saw in the images, and that they experience in their own lives.

FIFTEEN

Care ethics and physical restraint in residential childcare

Laura Steckley

Introduction

When social care workers must respond to behaviour which poses serious, imminent danger, the response can sometimes take the form of physical restraint. Physical restraint has long been the subject of serious concern in social care, as well as other areas, such as law enforcement and psychiatry. This chapter focuses on physical restraint in residential childcare. It is one of the most complex and ethically fraught areas of practice, yet there is almost no dedicated literature that applies itself to the ethical dimensions of this practice in this field. The chapter starts with discussion of the context of practice in residential childcare. A tentative explanation for and critique of the lack of ethically dedicated attention to the subject of physical restraint in residential childcare is then provided, with an argument for the transformative potential of care ethics to develop related thinking and practice. The chapter goes on to draw from a large-scale qualitative study of physical restraint in residential childcare in Scotland. The study was funded by Save the Children, Scotland and included in-depth interviews with 41 care workers and 37 children and young people. Interviews were comprised of four multi-level vignettes and a semi-structured interview schedule and averaged around 100 minutes for workers and 30 minutes for children and young people. Relevant findings are then examined and discussed through the lens of care ethics. While the contextual issues and findings discussed below are located specifically in Scotland, they have relevance to residential childcare (and indeed other forms of care where physical restraint is used) in the United Kingdom and internationally.

Context

In Scotland, residential childcare is comprised of a range of provision that includes secure accommodation, residential schools for children with emotional and behavioural difficulties, children's homes and homes that provide respite to families whose child or children are disabled. The vast majority of children and young people who are placed in residential care have experienced abuse, neglect and/or other trauma (Anglin, 2002; Ward, 2006) and sometimes their related, underlying pain can manifest in behaviours that pose risk of serious harm to themselves and/or others. According to the National Task Force on Violence Against Social Care Staff (2000), of those working in social care, practitioners who work with teenagers in residential care are one of the groups suffering the most violence, and it is children in their teenage years who are most represented in the residential childcare population (The Scottish Government, 2013).

There are particular complexities in these settings that impact on practice, and on the use of restraint specifically. They include: a continuing perception of residential childcare as a last-resort service (McPheat et al, 2007); the related practice of placing only children and young people with the most serious difficulties in residential care (Forrester, 2008); poor levels of workers' qualification, given the complex demands of the work (Heron, 2006); and the 'dark shadow' cast by the 'unremitting nature of the focus on institutional abuse' (Corby et al, 2001, p 181). As a result, care in residential childcare is carried out in a context that, at best, is ambivalent towards it.

Residential childcare is also affected by a wider social work context in which the central role of relationship has been significantly stifled by managerialism (Munro, 2011). The foundational principles of economy, efficiency and effectiveness (Audit Commission, 1993) upon which managerialism rests are derived from business models and are poorly suited to the context of helping professions (Meagher and Parton, 2004). They are based on 'an understanding of human behaviour that privileges cognition, rationality, and predictability and pays less attention to the emotional, irrational and unpredictable dimensions of human beings' (Ruch, 2011). Specific impacts of managerialism in residential childcare include an increased focus on outcomes, many of which are nonsensical in that the 'outcomes' for children who come from a long history of deprivation, abuse and/or other trauma – a long history often due to the residential care being used as a last resort – are being measured against the general population rather than children of similar histories (Forrester, 2008). It is the reparative experiences of care, relationship and self that are central to the healing potential of residential childcare, yet it can take a long time for these experiences to have an impact and, when they do, they are often not particularly measurable. There may indeed be an inverse relationship between what is important and what is easily measurable (Scottish Council Foundation, 1999).

Another key impact of managerialism is the framing of care in technical-rational terms. This can be seen in the raft of policies, procedures and paperwork now central to a residential childcare worker's task (Smith et al, 2013), as well as other technologies of care that include a variety of assessment tools and programmed interventions (Webb, 2006; Smith, 2009). Even care workers' reference to basic exchanges of touch have been found to use language of techniques derived from crisis-intervention training packages (Steckley, 2012). Finally, managerialist emphasis on governing the actions of front-line workers (Meagher and Parton, 2004) can be seen in the erosion of the authority of heads of residential homes and the diversion of decision-making power to external managers or health and safety personnel, many of whom have little understanding of the complexities and ambiguities of relationships in residential childcare (Smith, 2009).

The reductivist and simplifying impulses behind managerialism (Moss and Petrie, 2002; Smith, 2009) are not conducive to the highly complex and demanding nature of residential childcare work (Anglin, 2002; Ward, 2006; Garfat, 2008; Stevens, 2008; Steckley and Smith, 2011). Situations leading up to and involving the practice of physical restraint are one of the strongest illustrations of this demanding complexity. For the purposes of this chapter, physical restraint is defined as 'an intervention in which workers hold a child to restrict his or her movement and [which] should only be used to prevent harm' (Davidson et al, 2005, p viii). While there is a recent trend in some residential establishments towards calling restraints 'safe holds' (presumably based on the name of Scottish guidance), many restraints are experienced as violence by young people and by care workers (Steckley and Kendrick, 2008b). Negative effects can be severe and long lasting, not only on young people but also on the workers who carry them out. These can include physical injury, demoralisation, and trauma/re-traumatisation (Allen, 2008). Yet some efforts to avoid physical restraint, including the use of medication, seclusion or involvement of the police, have the potential to be even more damaging to young people and to their relationships with those who care for them (Steckley, 2009). Additionally, young people identify a need for physical restraint in situations of imminent or actual harm (Paterson et al, 2003; Steckley and Kendrick, 2008c; Morgan, 2012), and some young people have reported more positive effects of being restrained (Steckley and Kendrick, 2008c; Steckley, 2010).

Effective restraint reduction requires strong leadership and investment at almost all organisational levels, including staffing, training and development, unit culture, therapeutic approaches and, fundamentally, relationships (Fisher, 2003; Colton, 2004; Paterson et al, 2008). This has significant resource implications, as does the introduction of Snoezelen (Lancioni et al, 2002) or sensory rooms (Champagne and Stromberg, 2004) as alternatives to restraint. Such alternatives are becoming more prevalent in psychiatric settings or services for people with learning disabilities or dementia, but have yet to make an impact on the residential childcare sector (see Freeman, 2011, for a North American exception).

Ethics, residential childcare and physical restraint

Despite on-going concerns about the restraint of children and young people, there has been little written that provides an analysis of the related ethical dimensions of practice (Cornwall, 2006 and Wilkins, 2012 are two notable exceptions); still less has been theorised from an ethical or moral-philosophical perspective. There are several possible reasons for this lack of attention. Residential childcare has a relatively short history of research and scholarship as compared with, for example, medicine, where more has been written about the ethics of physical restraint from a bio-medical perspective (see, for example, Strumpf and Evans, 1991; Taxis, 2002; Gastmans and Milisen, 2006). In social work, within which residential childcare is professionally incorporated in the United Kingdom, the curricular requirement for dedicated ethics content in the honours degree has come about relatively recently (QAA, 2000; Department of Health, 2002). While some who work in residential childcare have completed the honours degree in social work, most workers currently achieve lower levels of qualification (Scottish Institute of Residential Child Care, 2010) – ones that do not require dedicated ethics curricula.

Dominant approaches to ethical theorising draw on traditions that locate moral deliberation in the public realm and emphasise a moral agent who applies ethical principles in a detached, impartial, rational and universal manner (Tronto, 1993). These approaches do not lend themselves to the complexities of providing personal care in a domestic setting that is simultaneously a public setting, subject to policies, regulation and inspection (Steckley and Smith, 2011).

Consequentialist arguments, crudely applied, can be used to justify poor practices related to physical restraint. Universal principles of imminent danger and last resort (criteria applied in assessing the acceptability of restraint) are widely supported (Day, 2000; Hart and Howell, 2004; Davidson et al, 2005), but in practice are ambiguous. Interpretations of what constitutes imminent danger or last resort can vary greatly, both in general and in the moment. Predicting the consequences of one course of action over another is not wholly reliable under ideal circumstances; in the lead-up to a physical restraint, with its complex, multiple variables and extreme emotional charge, these variances can be even more pronounced.

Rights-based discourses, drawing on a deontological tradition, have a dominant influence on policy and practice in residential childcare (Smith, 2009). Their development in Anglophone contexts has been predicated on the notion of contractual and/or legal mediation of relationships between individuals – individuals who are constructed as rational and autonomous (Dahlberg and Moss, 2005). Such an orientation can obscure the interdependent, affective and reciprocal nature of caring relationships and undermine the centrality of trust within them (Held, 2006). 'Trust is a quality often missing from simplistic conceptions of rights, which can distort thinking into adversarial terms (for example workers' rights versus young people's rights or rights versus responsibilities), stripping out the context and complexity of relationships' (Steckley and Smith, 2011, p 185).

The impacts of managerialism can make it difficult to hold on to the values and motivations that attract workers to social care in the first place (Moss and Petrie, 2002; Smith, 2009). Aronson and Smith (2010, 2011) describe social service managers' struggle to resist managerial practices that subvert their own professional values and the perceived precariousness of their 'valued selves' within their wider professional identity. Resistance, however, requires the perception that there is something that needs holding on to, and something to resist. The managerial tendency to reduce problems to technical and administrative issues obscures their ethical dimensions (Moss and Petrie, 2002). Ash (2010, p 205) identifies this tendency in her study of elder abuse, arguing that 'the social and political context of the work of social workers and their managers mitigated their alertness, or attentiveness, to barely acceptable situations for older people'. Bauman (2006) names this tendency adiaphorisation and argues that it leads to an ethical deskilling of workers by desensitising their moral sensibilities and repressing their moral urges. There was similar evidence of ethical deskilling and obscuring in the study, which will be discussed in the next section.

Care ethics offers not only a critique of traditional ethical approaches and the managerialist paradigm, but a framework against which care can be meaningfully and ethically assessed. It is an *ethic* of care, not simply care, that is needed (Held, 2006). Its fundamental project of making relational realities explicit (Gilligan, 1982) is highly relevant to residential childcare and the messy, complex work of cultivating close, caring relationships with children who have been relationally harmed. Its attention to context, particulars and emotion (Held, 2006) makes possible a meaningful engagement with the ambiguities of relational practice.

Care ethics provides a language that can enable discussions and debates that foreground and make sense of the ethical dimensions of practice (Barnes, 2012a). Shifts in language can reshape beliefs (Vojak, 2009), and the transformative potential of care ethics' language resides in its resonance with workers' experience and its ability to reignite their values. Moreover, care ethics' call to action on institutional and structural levels (Tronto, 1993, 2013) offers a means for envisaging residential childcare within a wider care system, one where determinations of resources, training and professional standing are no longer dominated by managerialist conceptualisations.

Findings

The first-level content analysis yielded a more subtle and complex account of the phenomenon of physical restraint than was previously reflected in the literature. Almost all respondents (workers, children and young people) indicated at some point in their interview that physical restraint was sometimes necessary and acceptable. They consistently connected its appropriate or acceptable use with issues of danger, destruction, risk, harm, safety or protection. There was also a dominant theme about the importance of attempting less-intrusive interventions and that restraint should be used only as a last resort. So while there was a general consensus across the majority of care workers and young people about the conditions under which restraint was seen as acceptable, further discussion exposed significant ambiguity about the degree and type of harm necessary to justify a restraint, the accuracy of assessments of the degree of harm and of imminence (especially under what were usually highly pressured and emotive conditions) and at what point other interventions should be abandoned and physical restraint should happen (again, this was the case for both workers and young people). From this, one can see the gross limitations of a technical-rational application of imminent harm and last resort, as well as the need for an ethical framework that engages with context, particulars and emotion.

All respondents recounted negative emotions and experiences of either being involved in a physical restraint or witnessing one (a very small number of respondents had only witnessed restraint). Some young people (around a third) also recounted positive experiences or effects of physical restraints, and some workers identified positive effects on young people. Experiences, both negative and almost all positive, were strongly linked to the perceived quality of the relationships among those involved – both before the restraint and subsequent to it. In other words, and in contrast to dominant related discourses (Steckley and Kendrick, 2008a), some young people recounted feeling safe, cared for or protected in/by the restraint, due to the safety and trust they felt for the workers involved; additionally, some young people stated that they felt more trust in workers due to the way a situation (in which restraint was a part) was handled. Conversely, some young people reported extremely negative experiences of restraint, based on poor relationships with those doing the restraining, and damage to relationships as a result of unnecessary or excessively rough restraints.

From a care ethics perspective, the findings related to relationships make sense. The perceived quality of a relationship would clearly impact on the degree to which a restraint was experienced as an act of care and protection, and the degree to which it was experienced as violence and coercion. Given the complex, ambiguous nature of situations involving restraint, it is often not a question of either/or: a heady and contradictory mix of powerful motivations and emotions can all be present in an incident involving restraint. Attending to relationship prior to, during and following incidents involving restraint will strongly influence which motivations and emotions dominate the experience and the subsequent meaning made of that experience. From a care ethics perspective, this attending (or the absence of it) is an ethical issue.

In the semi-structured interview schedule, workers were asked what ethical considerations affected their use of restraint. Their responses had a very different quality to other questions in the interview; well over half of the respondents visibly struggled to answer the question and a third clearly stated that they did not understand the question. Their discussion became unclear, at times even incoherent, and their discomfort was palpable. The adiaphorising impact of managerialism offers a potential way of understanding these reactions; many responses reflected an ethical deskilling, though the consistent, discernible emotional charge also present within their responses may belie a continued sensitisation to the ethical dimensions of physical restraint. It was as if there was an 'ethical stomach ache' related to this area of practice, but the words to articulate or make sense of it were lacking.

Well under a quarter of respondents did offer a clearer response to the question of ethical considerations. Their most frequently cited ethical consideration was related to whether the restraint was done for the right reasons and that it needed to be for the safety or protection of individuals involved. Misuse of power was most commonly commented on in terms of unethical use of restraint, though no respondent explicitly labelled it as such. Some stayed in clearly technical-rational territory, citing adherence to policy, procedure and risk assessments. Interestingly, no respondent made reference to their relationship with the child as an ethical consideration. Neither did any respondent speak of children's rights or a duty of care (current ethical lexicon applied to residential childcare) in response to the question. Children's rights and a duty of care did appear on a very few occasions elsewhere in interview, and it is interesting that these terms did not serve respondents when asked for their ethical considerations. It may well be that the language of duties and rights has not made its way more strongly into workers' thinking and language because the current managerialist context saps these concepts of their vitality in addressing more complex dimensions of practice.

Tacitly, most workers seemed aware that physical restraint is an ethically complex area of practice, and they raised significant, related concerns throughout their interviews. They discussed ambiguities of its practice, conveyed considerable ambivalence about its use and consistently expressed guilt, doubt and defeat for not being able to avoid it. At organisational levels, an over-reliance on technical-rational approaches appears to have obscured the ethical dimension of physical restraint. All of the establishments who participated in the study appeared to have policies and procedures in place related to physical restraint. A great deal of energy appears to have gone into training and refreshers, related paperwork (incident forms, debriefing forms) and requirements to inform families and social workers of occurrences of restraint (Steckley, 2010). There was, however, far less evidence of attention given to spaces for naming and making ethical sense of the complexities, ambiguities and anxieties related to the practice of restraint. For example, most workers described their experiences of debriefing (post restraint) as happening only 'in theory', inconsistently or superficially.

Discussion: physical restraint and care ethics?

Barnes (2012) argues that the development of ethical skills and sensibilities is required for care ethics potential to be realised, and this involves enabling processes and environments which foster workers' reflection on ethics. For this to be possible, workers need to see ethics not as policy or politics happening 'out there', but as relevant here and now (Ash, 2010). The conceptual orientation and language of care ethics hold promise for making this relevance accessible and real. For example, when workers and young people discussed the impacts of restraint on their relationships and vice versa, the language of care ethics was strongly reflected. They spoke of trust, understanding, need, dialogue, context, relationships and care (Gilligan, 1982; Noddings, 1984; Tronto, 1993; Parton, 2003; Held, 2006). Yet care workers did not consider their relationship with the young person as an ethical consideration related to restraint.

Care ethics' attention to care receiving (Tronto, 1993) highlights the importance of including the views and experiences of young people in the development of ethical skills and sensibilities of workers. Processes of naming and making sense among workers and young people are also served by the language of care ethics. Such processes contribute to the development of relationships that can hold episodes of imminent danger without recourse to physical restraint, or can provide the foundation for restraint to be experienced as an act of care if it does become necessary.

Restraint is portrayed as violence in much of the literature, and respondents' experiences reflect both violence and care. Held (2010, p 121) asserts that 'even in the context of care, violence may occasionally be called for ...The point of these uses of violence is to further the aims of care'. Held's quote offers a way in to understanding how a young person can describe her experience of restraint as feeling cared for, but close attention to power (Tronto, 2010) is necessary in order to determine whether such a restraint furthered the aims of care or further distorted the young person's understanding of caring relationships. Moreover, the way that power is enacted at all levels within an organisation, and not just within the confines of an incident and the relationships within it, must be considered. If the aims of care are to promote compensatory and healing relationships, relational congruence is necessary across all levels of the organisation (Anglin, 2002).

Does this mean that violence has a legitimate place in residential childcare practice? Certainly no respondent made such an explicit, bold statement. The aforementioned trend of calling a restraint a safe hold may indeed belie an underlying sense of the unacceptability of violence in the context of a caring institution, but it also has a euphemistic quality. Such distancing from the uncomfortable realities of physical restraint serves to repress related anxieties and inhibit processes of naming and making sense.

When workers enter a situation with a young person whose emotions and behaviours are escalating towards harm, and particularly at the point of initiating a restraint, it would be fair to say that they are demonstrating a willingness (albeit often an ambivalent and/or reluctant willingness) to potentially go to a violent place with that young person. In some cases, they may already be there. Is this the same thing as using violence to further the aims of care? It would be interesting to go back and ask worker respondents whether they felt they had 'used violence'. It is clear from the data that some young people felt that violence had been used against them; conversely, others did not – even when the restraint itself could have been characterised, at the very least, as coercive if not violent.

The integrated ability to hold on to the aims of care, in both one's activity and disposition (Tronto, 1993), through an episode involving restraint is of great importance in how the element of violence is experienced. In order for the relationship to hold and withstand the eruption of violence, workers must be able to convey unwavering care throughout the process; there must be congruence between their affect, actions and communication of care and last resort. Such relationships exemplify the kind courage and emotional stamina that continues to be insufficiently noted and valued (Gilligan, 1982).

Conclusion

Physical restraint must be understood within the context of relationships. The relational, emotional, embedded realities of situations involving restraint are far better served by care ethics, which attends to their relevance and puts relationship at the centre of its consideration. To develop safe, ethical and developmentally rich environments, residential cultures must make space for, and effectively address, related ambiguities and tensions, including those between care and control and the impact of violence on care environments. This can be particularly difficult in such an ethically fraught area of practice, but for this reason it is all the more necessary. If residential childcare is to truly attend to and meet the needs of children and young people who are in pain, then the relationships within this care must be able to hold the related complex, ambiguous, contentious dynamics and manifestations of that pain with ethical clarity. Care ethics offers a language and orientation that can facilitate such clarity and transform related practice.

SIXTEEN

Care for carers: care in the context of medical migration

Teodora Manea

Introduction

In March 2014, a 37-year-old Romanian anaesthesiologist killed herself in the French hospital where she was working. She left behind a six-year-old son and a loving husband. It does not seem that there were any problems in her personal life. However, she worked too hard. Her colleagues said she had to work 78 hours during the last week before her death and that she was drained and missed spending time with her family (Gervais, 2014). One day it all became too much for her and she ended her life. Her case is not exceptional. At first glance, doctors have the power and knowledge to bring other people's lives back on track, but they are also human beings who, when placed in a different context of life and work, will increasingly become more fragile, interdependent and in need of care.

Doctors as care givers are themselves a part of the complex web of care (Fisher and Tronto, 1990; Barnes, 2012a, p 40; Tronto, 2013, p 19) that connects individuals and families to each other and other members of society. In the case of migration, this web is torn apart as a result of the decision to move and the factors that may influence that decision. This may put migrant doctors in a different situation, in need of care themselves. To identify the care needs of migrant doctors I concentrate on three types of vulnerabilities connected to medical migration: professional, personal and socio-cultural.

Are migrant doctors privileged in comparison to other migrant workers? They are, after all, not 'illegal', and they receive a good salary that allows doctors to move to the destination country with their families and to not struggle with poverty. When I started an empirical study about medical migration from Romania to the UK (2010–14) I imagined that I would find people who would tell me about how having a well-paid job and a high social status in the UK had positively changed and enhanced their lives. But I discovered an unexpected range of social, professional and emotional problems, and people who were not well integrated and who were in need of care. Eastern European doctors are attracted to Western societies by a combination of *push* and *pull* factors such as better salaries and working conditions in the West, and poor salaries, difficult working condition, corruption and limited career opportunities in the country of origin. Most studies of medical migration analyse the decision to emigrate in terms of push and pull factors, but fail to acknowledge the long, hard and emotionally expensive process of adaptation to a new society (Dubois et al, 2006). The study revealed that the primary reason for doctors to emigrate was their unhappiness with Romanian society and their loss of hope and of trust that political reforms would be able to create better conditions for their work and living (Manea, 2011). Caring or less-caring societies (Held, 2006; Barnes, 2012a; Tronto, 2013) can be conceptualised as a further push/pull factor in migration.

The original research aimed to understand the conditions of migration in depth from the experiences of the doctors and their families, but this reflection of the need for care prompted me to examine this aspect of the doctors' lives in relation to an ethics of care. My intention is to draw attention to vulnerabilities from an ethics-of-care perspective. I will start my analysis by considering individual *autonomy* and interdependencies in the context of migration, and will then focus on three types of *vulnerability* – professional, personal and socio-cultural – that confront migrant doctors. Finally, I will challenge the idea of caring societies in connection with the healthcare market and care policies.

Individual autonomies and interdependencies in understanding migration

How could an ethic-of-care analysis inform an ethical discussion about medical migration? By placing the individual and the countries in the context of care relationships we can make duties, responsibilities and the motives for medical migration more concrete. In a dialectical way I emphasise that a person is situated *synchronically* in different care relationships, being at the same time care giver and care receiver. *Diachronically*, the relation of care is a reversible one during our lifetime: as children, as patients and as elderly, we need care. As adults we are expected to provide care for others. Our relation to a particular person (like a parent or a child) can switch from care receiver to care giver and vice versa. In the context of medical migration, this dialectic sheds light on the synchronic care relationships that migrant doctors are involved in: caring *for* and *about* patients and families, receiving care and support from their family, being in need of social care in the origin and destination countries. The diachronic perspective highlights how the social construction of migrant doctors as 'healthcare workforce' ignores their life span, by isolating only the active working life needed for the care market, such that the duty for education of children and for the care of the elderly is ignored (Berger and Mohr, 2010).

Migration pulls individuals away from their usual synchronic care relationships and alters the balance of their web of care. Paradoxically, while it is intended to be a remedy to existing difficulties faced by the migrant in the home country, migration creates new challenges. To make visible the existential dimension of migration it is worth reflecting on the concepts of individual choice and responsibility. Is migration really just a matter of individual choice to change one's life? It may seem as if an autonomous individual had made a rational choice for which they now bear moral responsibility. Thus, emigrating doctors are blamed in the countries of origin for the ensuing brain drain and for endangering the right to health of their own fellow citizens (Plotnikova, 2012). From the perspective of the destination countries, they bear responsibility for their failure or success in cultural adaptation. In this way, the responsibilities of both origin and destination countries for migration are ignored, and the discourse is focused on individual responsibility (Tache and Schillinger, 2009). This individualistic perspective overlooks the international extent of responsibilities for care migration and diminishes the decisional factors and the relational ontology (Barnes, 2012a, pp 11–13) of human beings. If we change the equation: individual–*autonomy*–choice–responsibility to cluster–*web of care*–vulnerability–care, the landscape of migration will look different.

That a doctor is seen as a rational, independent agent able to look at the pros and cons of migration and to make a decision, a choice, on a presumed autonomy is highly questionable (Fineman, 2004; Barnes, 2012a). The migrant doctors I interviewed came to the UK for and with their families. The economic difficulties affecting the whole family, and the need to care for one's children, were important push factors in leaving Romania in order to achieve a better life for them. At the same time this created a huge responsibility.

> "There is a huge responsibility to go with the whole family, but the needs are pushing you. I was tired and scared. I was scared that I'll be ill someday and not able to work

and pay back the loans. I had to go. I had to pay back the loans." (Horia)

This doctor was part of a web of care: for his children and wife, care for the patients in the UK, care for his mother left in Romania – and he cared for his country of origin as well. He was diagnosed with thyroid cancer, so he was a patient himself, vulnerable and scared. He tried to ensure a future for his two young children.

We live in complicated *clusters* of ties, loves, needs, vulnerabilities; we share moral, familial or social depth with others. The feeling of being part of a certain community or family determines the degree of our freedom and our choice. The doctors in this study experienced sometimes conflicting needs, interests and obligations to themselves and others. An ethic of care recognises the complex personal and social contexts within which individuals make decisions, and the significance of care as a motivator for such decisions.

For doctors, responsibility for care in the public domain has a double aspect: to care for your own society, as a personal environment where you feel 'at home', and to care for the members of this society as potential patients or people in need of care. But the socioeconomic context affects the social responsibility of doctors in terms of care. The doctors I interviewed told me that, in Romania, miserable salaries endanger the functioning of the household. Many young doctors could not afford to have their own accommodation. In one case, a young family of three were sharing a two-bedroomed apartment with their parents and another brother. One doctor recalled times when he couldn't afford to buy nappies for his child. In many cases, a deprived household is the first motive underpinning the decision to emigrate. The moral principle underlying this attitude can be best described as: 'care for your *next!*', which has more moral power than 'care for society!', especially when that society is not perceived as supportive. The doctors told me that they felt like they had a moral duty to care for their families first. Some may argue that caring for your own children may be a case of what Tronto has referred to as a care pass 'Only my Own' (Tronto, 2013, pp 175–7). But those children are not going to be part of a special-status group; on the contrary, they will share the status of 'migrant children' in the destination countries.

Types of vulnerability

It is hard to justify the need of care where one cannot see any vulnerability. Assessing vulnerabilities should precede the discourse about care needs, responsibilities, resources and allocation, because our views about what we consider *vulnerable* determine our moral action and responsibility in providing care. Vulnerability defines an exposed part of a human being, a space endangered by potential harm. Migration is a way of life for an increasing number of people in the 21st century. The internet, social media and affordable travel make our lives mobile and fluid. But facilitators of migration are not necessarily facilitators of integration into a new socio-cultural environment. Migration is a double *othering* process, first because one's 'home' is left behind; and second because the migrant is now living in the home of the others. Strangers are 'outsiders' to a community, and the orientation and integration into a new world come with a cost. This is not calculated or seen when highly skilled medical migration is understood from the perspective of its economic mechanisms. Decent UK salaries may compensate for the vulnerability caused by material insecurity (needs and debts), but not, for example, professional and personal vulnerabilities.

Professional vulnerability

We do not normally think of doctors as vulnerable, because usually our care-oriented attention is directed to the patient. But the medical profession, despite its high social status and good money, has an emotionally consuming price. A US study (Miller and Mcgowen, 2000) showed that the suicide rate among doctors has been between 28 and 40 per 100,000, compared with the rate in the general population of 12.3 per 100,000. To psychological problems connected with the medical profession, the fact of being a migrant adds more difficulties: medical language and communication with patients from another culture, different names for drugs, different institutional ways and regulations. The medical profession combines the *power* of the doctor with the representation and expectation of intimate *care* (Gilligan and Pollak, 1988). Both are culturally embedded and rely on trust (Helman, 2007). Doctors generally can find themselves between two distinct vulnerabilities. Firstly, the intimate relation with the patient may affect the objectivity of practice and diagnosis. Secondly, the permanent need for perfection of the knowledge and skills necessary for a medical career may distance the doctor from human relationships and isolate them. Ethical codes, training programmes and professional texts are meant to secure the objectivity of medical practice. But the more subtle danger of isolation is not problematised to the same extent (Gilligan and Pollak, 1988, p 245). According to Gilligan and Pollak, there seems to be a gender-specific reaction to those two vulnerabilities: men associated danger with *intimacy* and women saw more danger in *impersonal* achievement and *isolation* associated with competitive success. My interviewees also spoke of family sacrifices:

> "There is a moment when it is hard, especially if you have family and children and there is this and that still to be done. You finish your training but there is still something to learn and it's hard to impose sacrifices on the others, to make them believe in your dreams" (Ioan)

Migrant doctors have to face the vulnerability of *understanding*, both understanding the patient and understanding how institutions function. The last vulnerability is being remote from your own country, not having the network of friends and family for help in difficult moments, and not completely understanding the way a society and a culture are structured and function. One interviewee summarised it like this:

> "There is incertitude of two kinds. One is that of a man who leaves behind his family, his world, his country, his friends, everything that is familiar and that makes your life easier. And the profession you somehow knew (...) everything goes. And what is more, you have an uncertainty connected to the way you practise medicine here." (Ioan)

Another doctor reflected anxiety about communication with patients:

> "At the beginning you are scared, you don't know what to tell (the patients), if you can tell this and that. We were warned that the Romanians and Germans were too direct ..." (Maria)

Understanding patients does not merely require a good level of English. In order to address a question, to communicate a diagnosis, or sometimes to perform a simple medical act, a doctor needs to know how the psychology of this particular patient works. The act of care implies *trust*. If the patient feels a doctor's hesitation, some cultural discomfort – due to insufficient knowledge about cultural codes – or some kind of aggressive paternalism, the trust building and therefore the care process may become compromised. Compared to the UK, Romanian society includes few minority ethnic groups, except Roma.

For a doctor coming to the UK for the first time, Indian, Pakistani, Caribbean or African cultures are completely new and unknown territory. One of my interviewees reflected uncertainty about relating to patients from different cultural backgrounds: "you don't know what these patients expect from you, how they imagine what is a good doctor" (Irina).

There is an asymmetry between Eastern and Western Europe regarding the structure, role and functions of 'caring institutions' (Tronto, 2013). This is based on different social histories, and although the capitalist model of care as a commodity to be purchased (Barnes, 2012a, p 69) is increasingly evident in Eastern Europe, one of the interviewed dentists complained that his patients regard the doctor–patient interaction in terms of a supermarket and undermine his professional advice:

> "They want something, and you try to explain to them
> that it is not feasible because of anatomical or physiological
> particularities, but they insist. 'I pay, you do it', like in a
> supermarket ..." (Horia)

This conflicts with a paternalistic model of doctor power that is still present in Romania (Teodorescu et al, 2013). Cultural barriers like language, stereotypes, behavioural and professional norms can generate frustration or lack of trust for both patients and doctors. The principles of care ethics articulated by Tronto (1993): attentiveness, responsibility, competence, responsiveness; trust (Sevenhuijsen, 1998) and respect (Engster, 2007) may be understood and practised differently in different cultural contexts. If the care givers and the care receivers were socialised in different cultures, personal representation of care may be affected by different cultural stereotypes (Lister et al, 2007; Williams and Gavanas, 2008; Williams, 2010).

Back in Romania, the Romanian doctors who were interviewed spoke of the professional and moral problems generated by small salaries that may put doctors in the humiliating corruption chain:

> "In Romania you are not treated with respect as a doctor,
> you don't have the dignity you deserve ... the general
> opinion in Romania is that the doctors are corrupt with
> small salaries, but they can manage it, because they put their
> hands in our pockets." (Irina)

Doctors spoke about the frustration of not being able to do their job:

> "It is inhuman and embarrassing to ask ill people to bring their own medicine so that you can treat them. I couldn't stay there and ask the patients to come with gloves, bandages and everything from home in order to receive a more or less correct medical treatment." (Irina)

A negative mass media image of doctors in Romania (medical errors are easily turned into media headlines); the indifference of politicians regarding the reform and function of the healthcare system; and some more objective facts such as total expenditure on health of 5.4% of GDP in 2008, as compared to 8.7% in the UK, all create the image of a less caring society. This may weaken the sense of responsibility felt by the doctor in a country that has invested insufficient resources in healthcare.

Personal vulnerability

Five interviewees spoke of tensions generated by a partner who could not find or afford work in the UK because of childcare duties. The costs of childcare in the UK and the absence of the extended family force doctors' partners to undertake the care work at home. For those accustomed to undertaking paid work, the new situation of 'staying at home' is perceived as a dependent, unworthy one. This fact is a consequence of the contrasting *work* versus *care culture* (Barnes, 2012a; Tronto, 2013). In the study of participant-observed couples, the partners were willing to undertake even a very low-status job – as cleaners, drivers or caretakers – just to avoid the isolation and the frustration of being at home. It is hard to explain why this phenomenon occurs in terms of 'rationality' of the individual. The money made from these activities was less than the money spent for replacement childcare. Why do people not want to stay at home with their children, reading books and enjoying long walks in the park? One answer may be that our identities are tailored by our interactions with *public* life. The absence of *public* life, accessible in the case of emigrants mainly via *work*, undermines personal identity. The *private* life is an insufficient source of identity. Being a wife or a husband *of a doctor* is not an acceptable social status for the highly skilled migrants accompanying them. Their decision to emigrate was driven by ideas of freedom and emancipation that conflict with the low social status of 'full-time mum' or 'caring, but not *working* dad'. Two of the couples

I studied separated as a result, and partners returned to Romania to resume their previous jobs. In one case the children returned with the partner, so that the doctor working in the UK remained there solely to meet the family's economic needs.

The migrant doctors and their partners described frequently feeling lonely and isolated. The previous social network of friends and extended family was not rebuilt in the UK, so they complained of a lack of emotional support. The feeling of being alone was accentuated by the representation of their 'social future'. It was striking that nearly all participants in this study dreamed of a retirement in Romania, although social protection of the older population there is still poor. But somehow the subjective and personal comfort of being with their own people seems to be much stronger. The representation of becoming more frail and vulnerable with age and 'having to die amongst strangers' made them long for the return to their country of origin. They want to share the vulnerability of age with their friends and extended family, rather than to experience it among strangers. The financial profit made by working abroad will be transformed into a personal bubble of social security.

Socio-cultural vulnerability

Socio-cultural vulnerability is understood as an umbrella concept for all problems caused by interactions with a new environment; particularly the expression of self and the understanding of the others in form of language, customs and physical appearance. For migrant, who has their own culturally specific constructions (such as the belief that education in the UK generally means something of the quality provided by institutions like Oxford and Cambridge), even the most trivial things can become a massive challenge, if not an ordeal. Even after integrating themselves to a certain point into the new culture, the vulnerability connected with incertitude and problematic identity continues:

> "You are the first migrant generation and you are not really integrated. Neither in the country (Romania) nor somewhere else ... What you (still) have is only the language and some people you know, but you are like 'neither horse nor donkey'." (Ioan)

The discomfort generated by cultural and personal identity is augmented with particular constructions of citizenship. As EU citizens, the Romanian doctors enjoy freedom of movement, and their qualification is formally recognised within the EU. However, Romanian and Bulgarian citizens, although part of the EU, have a negative social image as coming from two of the poorest EU countries. This fact is used in xenophobic public discourses that form the public image of these citizens (BBC, 2013b, 2013c). The negative social image of 'Romanians and Bulgarians' who come to the UK to abuse the benefit system (Davies and Malik, 2014) makes the Romanian doctors and their family members uncomfortable with their ethnicity. This may not affect doctors directly, as they are quite well regarded as professionals, but will affect their family members, either via discriminatory employment policies or by accentuating the feeling of social exclusion, 'othering' (Barnes, 2012a, p 114) and marginalisation. A diffuse process of self-exclusion, based on vulnerability resulting from the burdens of citizenship, may be used as a strategy to avoid rejection. They want to be *respected* for what they are and do as a *person*, they want *recognition* (Honneth, 1995) and not to be discriminated against as citizens of a country they have left. Job fairs and internet websites stimulate medical migration into the UK (NHS, 2013), in contrast to the public discourse against Romanian and Bulgarian emigrants who would 'invade' Britain to abuse the benefits system (BBC, 2013a). The national identity of Romanian doctors is affected by the image of what is publicly portrayed as 'being Romanian'.

Caring societies: healthcare market and care policies

The healthcare workforce is subject to market mechanisms in the same way as other workforces. As Tronto (2013, pp 114–15) emphasises, there are good and bad aspects of the care market generally. The market may show the *value* of care, and therefore underline the reality and importance of it. But the danger of viewing care only in market terms creates a distorted view of what care is and how caring responsibilities should be allocated. My argument is that health workers should not be subjected to market mechanisms in the same way that other human resources are, for two reasons: because of the international injustice that this creates (poor countries cannot meet their healthcare needs), and because the cultural aspects of healthcare are ignored. Those two aspects are neglected in healthcare and social policies.

The social protection of the population, especially regarding the delivery and management of healthcare, fails if the medical workforce is lost. But this is not just an issue for healthcare in the context of an ageing society. The local medical workforce in Western countries is insufficient to cover healthcare needs and to deal with what

Sevenhuijsen called the *relocation of care* in the medical world from *cure* to *care* (Sevenhuijsen, 2003, p 16). The political solution to 'import' doctors and other medical personnel who have been trained abroad can be considered careless. The duty of a social policy is more than to identify those people in need of care in Western Europe and to encourage migrant doctors to cover this need. The 'care deficit' (Tronto 2013) of ageing and welfare societies is not simply to be *covered* by workforce from other countries. The dislocation of care from one country to another creates new unmet needs of care resulting from 'global care chains' (Yeates, 2004; Hochschild, 2000; Williams, 2010). In relation to migrant doctors, this intra-European global *doctors'* care chain involves highly skilled migrants, with the implication not only of care displacement but also that the costs of medical education fall to those EU countries least able to afford them. Instead of managing care, medical migration will actually transfer the 'care deficit' to those who are least powerful within global socioeconomic relations.

Responses to this require political action. The EU Recognition of Professional Qualifications Directive, 2005/36/EC, 2006/100/CE and other international policies (World Bank, International Monetary Fund) (Tache and Schillinger, 2009) have encouraged the migration of doctors. Recruitment codes (NHS, 2004; WHO, 2011) aim to protect poorer countries from losing their doctors (Manea, 2011; Cehan and Manea, 2012), but these have no obligatory force (Wiskow, 2005). The UK's health and education policies should be questioned regarding inadequate provision of 'home-grown' doctors. According to the GMC report (2013), 39% of doctors on the Specialist Register have qualified outside the UK (GMC, 2013, pp 23–7). To import them is a cheaper alternative to training doctors at home, but is this a fair one? It is not fair to patients, who will face the difficulties of cross-cultural communication (Skelton et al, 2001), it is not fair to those UK students who want to study medicine, and it is not fair to the states that will lose this social resource.

Rather than thinking in terms of *health expenditure*, the ethics-of-care perspective suggests that money for health should be seen as an *investment* in a healthy society. Healthcare and education are, *par excellence*, investments for a healthy and efficient society – if we wish to stay with the economic way of thinking. The governmental discourse of 'health expenditure' has transformed healthcare into a service offered to population, a commodity. In terms of costs and supplies, foreign doctors are on the level of cheap supplies. This discourse collides with a view of healthcare as a fundamental human right. As this chapter has suggested, we need to think of this beyond national boundaries: are healthcare workers an important social resource, or just 'workers' on an international job market, part of the global movement of labour?

Conclusion

The ethics-of-care approach to understanding the moralities involved in medical migration highlights the vulnerabilities of doctors before and after the decision to emigrate. This may offer a better comprehension of migration mechanisms, beyond the 'push/pull' model. Migration from the origin country is a form of protest against the socioeconomic policies in place, and also a manifestation of mistrust regarding the local political capacity to change things in a foreseeable future. But going to another country does not automatically provide a new citizenship or make the migrant part of the new society. New social rules, new civil rights and obligations need to be learned, accepted and internalised. So the migrant doctors are twice deprived of their citizenship, of their socio-political web, and that fact feeds existential vulnerabilities such as insecurity, fear, isolation, alienation and marginalisation.

The key point in this chapter is that doctors are a social resource that needs to be cared *about* and cared *for* (Tronto, 2013) and the care deficit of a society should not be stated in purely economic terms and covered with an imported 'workforce'. The specificities of medical practice and its cultural embedding need to be considered from the perspective not only of medical migration policies but also of the general EU design of medical education.

SEVENTEEN

Mental health service use and the ethics of care: in pursuit of justice

Tula Brannelly

The issues of care and justice in mental health

Many chapters of this book have attended to the potential renewal offered by the ethics of care in various realms of everyday life. Here I use the ethics of care to address care in mental health services by drawing on data from a small qualitative research project. Justice and care are intertwined in the ethics of care, where achieving social justice requires relational care (Barnes and Brannelly, 2008). Two key aspects of the ethics of care make the analysis of justice and care possible. First, justice requires that practices are seen so that they may be judged (Tronto, 2013). As practices associated with detention and compulsion are 'hidden', in that they are largely unknown to people not connected to them, to be able to judge them requires that these practices are surfaced. Second, Tronto's (1993 and 2013) phases of care provide an analytical tool for the analysis of research data, and also, importantly, a position from which to renew care. First it is necessary to take a brief overview of the territory in which care is attempted in the context of mental health. My focus here is on policy and practice in the UK and New Zealand, which have similar mental health policy, legislation and services.

Every society has responses to care for people in need. But in the case of people with mental health problems particular responses are invoked that differentiate them as a group from others considered 'needy'. Deeply entrenched normative values operate to marginalise people who experience long-term mental illness. Societies that value productive, consuming citizens often reinforce the 'otherness' associated with mental illness. People with mental illness are marginalised and excluded on many levels. Acknowledging inequality for a particular group of people surfaces issues related to it, stated by Tronto (2013, p 91 quoting from Hirschmann, 2002, p 231):

> For instance, if a society repeatedly, systematically constrains women more than men, blacks more than whites, lesbians more than heterosexuals, then there is a theoretical presumption in favour of the conclusion that the society – or the rules, norms, institutions, practices, and values in question in a particular context where freedom is at issue – presents a barrier to the more constrained group.

Tronto (2013) highlights the need to pay attention to the experiences of particular groups in terms of inequality and care, and reminds us that rights, in the tradition of T.H. Marshall (1950), were never intended to meet the needs of people who are vulnerable.

People who use mental health services may do so voluntarily or be compelled to do so through legislation. Compulsion is used when individuals are considered to meet clinical criteria for risk or danger as a result of mental illness and do not concur with the need for service intervention. The criteria for the use of the Mental Health Act, and subsequent compulsion, are a diagnosable mental illness and risk of harm or self-neglect, or a risk of harm towards others as assessed by mental health clinicians (psychiatrists, nurses and social workers) who are given powers under legislation. The notions of risk and mental illness are contestable.

Where a person is assessed to fulfil the criteria of the Act, human rights may be overridden, justified by the need for protection of the person or others. Protection includes detention and compulsory treatment such as medications, and also the use of seclusion and restraint. When a person is detained, compulsion, restraint and seclusion may be used, human rights are contravened (Drew et al, 2011) and treatment can be given without consent. Compulsion can extend from the in-patient setting into the community through the use of community treatment orders. If human rights that constitute the taken-for-granted ascription of citizenship are removed, then the attribution of citizenship per se is, in practice, conditional on mental state as defined by clinical services. Individual 'rights to' are eclipsed by institutional 'control of' and 'control of' is often experienced as oppression (Owen and Floyd, 2010).

There may be many opportunities for practices that limit the disempowerment experienced by users of mental health services, such as maintaining levels of choice and control and offering services that meet people's preferences. Examples may include the avoidance of restraint, especially for people who have been subject to previous physical or emotional abuse, and that particular treatments, such as electroconvulsive therapy, are only ever given with consent. Practices are opportunities for examination of the use of power, care, control and citizenship. I have argued elsewhere that consideration of a permanent or temporary loss of autonomy, while retaining commitment to the values of citizenship and participation in care, requires a practice grounded in care ethics (see Brannelly, 2006, 2010, 2011).

Many problems have been noted regarding the implementation of mental health legislation. First, the spirit of the legislation was intended to provide protection to people in situations of crisis. However, in practice the use of compulsion has extended into long-term restrictions in far-reaching aspects of people's lives (Rugkasa and Burns, 2009). Second, the expectation is that people who are subject to detention and compulsion will be given proper treatment to improve their mental state. However, high levels of dissatisfaction with services and ineffective treatments persist. Third, although legislation also confers rights such as the right to review of detention, few instances of review find in favour of the person challenging this. Fourth, mental health service practices are largely 'hidden'. Those unconnected to them personally or professionally are unaware of what happens to people subject to compulsion, yet the use of such powers is accepted as a public benefit.

In a context in which increasing aspects of 'abnormality' are recorded as criteria for mental illnesses, large proportions of the population meet criteria for diagnosis. A recent community survey of mental health in Aotearoa New Zealand (ANZ) (Oakley Browne, Wells and Scott, 2006) identified that 20% of the population meet diagnostic criteria for a mental illness at any one time. In this country with a population of approximately 4.5 million, in 2012, 4,328 people were detained under the Mental Health Act on in-patient orders or on community treatment orders and 882 people were secluded while in care (Ministry of Health, 2013, p 14). According to the Health and Social Care Information Centre, in 2013 in England 22,000 people were detained and treated under the Mental Health Act or on a supervised community treatment order. In Western countries, about 3% of the population are diagnosed with a mental illness described as 'severe and enduring' or 'serious' with significant impacts on social inclusion and physical health. Among those with a diagnosis, levels of unemployment are as high as 80%, with poverty and poor housing common. A shortened life span is attributable to psychiatric medications and poor physical healthcare (Craig, 2008). Compulsory assessment and treatment is more often used with already marginalised populations such as Irish and Black people in England, Māori and Pacific peoples in ANZ. Māori constitute 14% of the population of ANZ, but 32% of seclusion events involved Māori patients (Ministry of Health, 2013). Such data questions evidence of a collective commitment to ensure justice and well-being for all citizens.

Spheres of 'hidden' work require scrutiny to inform collective responsibility. Independent scrutineers such as the Mental Health Act Commission in the UK and OPCAT, part of the Human Rights Commission, have at different times had a crucial role to inform governing bodies of human rights abuses and concerns. But such scrutiny is only part of what is necessary for justice. Also it is necessary to know the conditions and context for the loss of rights of some citizens, as this enables analysis of what can be considered protection and care (Tronto, 1993). Scrutiny is required so that society can judge the morality of these actions (Tronto, 2013).

Narrow procedural conceptions of justice focusing on the process of implementation of the Act, and an individual's right to redress through reviews that consider whether the criteria for detention and treatment have been met, are inadequate to achieving socially just responses to people experiencing severe mental health problems. Such a narrow reading of justice is unable to consider wider implications of inequality and marginalisation deriving from stigmatisation and discrimination. Recognition of systematic marginalisation calls for examination of the treatment of people with mental illness from a social justice perspective that also recognises the importance of care.

Emphasis on interdependencies in the ethics of care calls for a universal acceptance of vulnerability and challenges the marginalisation associated with dependence and need. This may help to decrease the 'otherness' associated with stigmatised and discriminated-against groups. Inequality in the ethics of care examines the positioning and treatment of certain groups in society and the particular contexts in which certain groups are constrained (Tronto, 2013, p 91). Tronto (2013, p 33) suggests that unquestioned protections remove political questions from public consideration. The conditions and contexts of protection are worthy of examination in terms of care:

> If protection is a form of care, then a set of questions about protection arise from the standpoint of a democratic caring society. If care concerns needs, who determines the needs for protection? And protection is 'protection from whom'? Iris Marion Young (2003) argued that there is a great danger if citizens simply accept the story about their need for protection and do not question it. (Tronto, 2013, p 75)

This quotation relates to the protections required from the threat from terrorism, but the same questions can be asked in this context of mental health services. Protection is often discussed in relation to a 'public' threat from a person 'out of control' or the need to protect a person from themselves.

Barnes (2012a, p 7) helpfully critiqued how policy and practice has come to constitute independence as 'choice and control' or dependence as 'care and protection'. This dyadic notion of care renders the care receiver as either able to choose and having control, or unable to choose and requiring protection. But of course, people may both be in need of care and protection and want choice and control.

Unseen or hidden practices cannot be judged. Public examination of practices regarding the use of mental health legislation should consider whether these can be understood as embodying care, an attempt at care or a lack of care. Applying the ethics-of-care phases as an analysis to data that examines the concerns of people who have experience of service use will help to answer these questions.

A small qualitative research project was undertaken in England and ANZ about 'acts of citizenship' (Isin, 2008). This research is part of my broader concern for citizenship and care that considers the experiences of people with mental health problems in relation to citizenship as a practice (Lewis, 1998) and status (Lister, 2003; Lanoix, 2007; Hart, 2009), and to understand what responses impede or sustain citizenship (Busfield, 2010). The 'acts of citizenship' research project was driven by a curiosity to know what people who have used services would consider the main issues that require change in mental health service provision. This curiosity evolved as a response to conversations with mental health service users in research and teaching.

Participants were involved in the service user/survivor movement, described here as 'service user activists', although some may not refer to themselves as such. I have used the term activist, as all participants were engaged in activities to promote change in mental health services, for example through governance, belonging to service user organisations and/or working as advocates. In the interviews, participants were asked to consider what key areas of change they thought were required in mental health service provision. There were three participants in England and six in ANZ and they were recruited through service user networks and interviewed in 2011 and 2012. Two of the nine participants were men. One participant asked to respond by e-mail. Pseudonyms are used for the research participants.

Participants drew on their various roles as family members, (ex) service users, advocates, educators, researchers, campaigners, peer service providers, mental health commissioners and network leaders. They welcomed the opportunity to discuss their concerns rather than the usual requests for consultation to respond to government agencies. While mental health policy prioritises easier access and greater choice in mental health services, participants referred to their own and others' experiences of detention, compulsion and force and prioritised these for the transformation of services.

Renewing care and justice with the ethics of care

In this presentation of analysis, data is presented that uncovers 'hidden' practices aligned with the five spheres of care (Tronto, 2013, pp 22–3), with a focus on solidarity, trust and relational care.

Caring about.

At this first phase of care, someone or some group notices unmet caring needs. Attentiveness.

People in distress are often part of care networks, although some may well be very isolated and excluded from their existing care networks. Professional help is sought when care within usual networks cannot be sustained. This is sometimes because on-going high levels of distress can be very difficult to cope with, and family members may themselves experience distress. Whatever the situation that care workers are invited into, it is their responsibility to understand what is working and what is not for the people within the care network.

The decision to invite paid workers into a care network is a significant step, an invitation to 'join with' the care that is already occurring. Recognition of the needs of all involved enables a negotiation to take place. Tensions, conflicts and difference may be present here, and the negotiation needs to be facilitated with this in mind. The voice of the person who requires protection needs to be heard, as this may inform the care process about whether protection is welcome or unwanted. Recognition of the person's preferences, needs and strengths in this way ensures that abilities and challenges are known and that the person is able to contribute where possible. A focus on 'care and protection' shifts the power away from the person, and their diverse strengths, abilities and needs may not be fully understood.

The lead into service use is often at a time of crisis when people are struggling to maintain themselves in their world. Fiona discussed what she found helpful in such a situation and what she advocated for on behalf of others:

"there are two things that are really helpful – it is great to have home treatment teams – I had to fight for that. Also it is essential to be able to define your own crisis and self-refer to crisis resolution."

Participants described their difficulty with understanding the purpose or the intent of the service, as they did not think that their needs or family needs were understood or valued. Lizzie critiqued services for missing the opportunity of helping her to make sense of what was happening for her:

"The other big question that they had no idea about helping me to answer was 'what's the meaning of this distress'. There was no interest in it, they just wanted to eradicate it."

Services defined people by their distress, and failed to link that distress to other aspects of the person's life, such as trauma. No attempts were made to understand how the person experienced their distress, or how they interpreted it. Service users were considered 'difficult' when they did not accept the assessment, diagnosis or treatments on offer. Assessments and treatment plans failed to understand what the person wanted from the service, as they did not ask what was important to the person. Lacking insight into illness was a term used where people did not see themselves as ill, or did not want medication. Where services failed to understand needs and respond effectively to them, the problem was located with the service user. Ellie:

"I've been called chronic, complex, severe, urgent, non-compliant, acute, treatment-resistant, long term.... and all by the time I was 24 years old."

Participants discussed a lack of acknowledgement of needs at different stages of using services. Teresa was told by the community service that she met its criteria for recovery and no longer required a service, despite having used it for over 20 years:

"And I have been told that I have recovered, that I am now well, and that if I need to go back to services I can but, you know, only in crisis sort of thing. And it may seem daft that someone like me, who has you know, speaks up and speaks out about mental health services, it is really hard to speak out about helping and help for yourself."

If services are not attentive to the people who use services, subsequent resources are misplaced and wasted. Also, systematic exclusion of the person, their experience and knowledge is neglectful and compounds distress. Enacting care becomes immediately impossible.

Caring for

Once needs are identified, someone or some group has to take responsibility to make certain that these needs are met.

In the ethics of care, responsibility is a call to action based on needs identified through attentiveness. Responsibility is therefore forward looking and based in action. Professional responsibility may be differently conceptualised as duty or obligation, and services may assume that families have obligations to meet needs. Families may want to take some responsibility, but may not be factored into care provision by services. Responsibility is action orientated and relational in care ethics, where opportunities for responsibility are recognised.

Services may not be able to meet needs considered beyond their remit. Few 'out of hours' services exist for people in distress and crisis, so people access hospital emergency departments as a place of safety or when injured. Attendance at a health provider is an opportunity for a potentially life-saving intervention, such as the prevention of a suicide. However, participants discussed how staff lacked responsibility to provide care. Ellie said:

> "I would say a lot of work needs to be done with emergency staff and police, particularly A&E (accident and emergency) staff to improve attitudes and decrease the stigma and discrimination which leads to some appalling mistreatment – which then leads to people not using those services when they need to, which is quite dangerous."

Participants discussed how poor attitudes prevailed, such as blame and being made to feel unwelcome in services.

Care-giving

The third phase of caring requires that the actual care-giving work be done. Competence.

In the ethics of care, competence relates to the ability to meet needs and having the necessary resources. Competence to provide care when people are in distress requires a connection between people so that distress is not exacerbated by isolation. Josephine spoke about her most recent experience of detention:

> "And distress or kind of mind chaos, however you want to frame the experience, people need things that [pause] they do not need to be shut off from other human beings. It just seems so simple to me.... So I might be a bit kind of high and not eat for three days, but eventually with some other kind of encouragement to rest and be nurtured with good food and sleep, I'm going to come out of that ..."

Competent care requires appropriate resources. Legislation was discussed as a way to guarantee access to limited service provision:

> "One of the conflations that happens in this debate is that people associate compulsory treatment with reliable services. So they think if we didn't have that [legislation] there, my relative would be neglected." (Lizzie)

People who ask for help expect competent services. Research participants recognised that family members did not always want the sort of help on offer from services. Ellie reflected on experiences of family members caring for people in rural and remote areas where services are inaccessible:

> "Families are often doing good work helping their family and need encouragement to continue that and reinforce that they are doing well. Currently, they tend to think that someone will step in and take control but they are not always pleased with the outcome when people do."

The way that care was currently being provided was often ignored, which meant that service providers did not join with care, but saw themselves as the primary care givers, ignoring the strengths and preferences of the care network (see Barnes, Chapter Three in this volume). Service users and care givers often want to be listened to, reassured and to receive practical help, which is demoted by the service focus on risks, safety and containment.

Care receiving

Once care work is done, there will be a response from the person, thing, group, animal, plant or environment that has been cared for. Observing that response and making judgements about it (for example, was the care sufficient?, successful?, complete?) is the fourth phase of care. Responsiveness.

Responsiveness requires that care providers are open to the responses of people who use services at individual, family and systemic levels. Mental health service user involvement is expected to inform and improve service provision. Some participants acted in senior governance roles to inform research funding, policy making and service provision as a representative of service user networks, or in a consultancy capacity. But participants noted fluctuating commitment to user involvement.

> "It is a sign of the times as well that the kind of expertise that they want in these power circles is not the kind that I have. They don't want any kind of service user expertise. The tide has gone out." (Lizzie)

Abdul identified the absence of an independent body to hear complaints, thereby making the process for change inadequate:

> "What is said about support for mental health and what you actually get is a big difference. If you complain you are complaining to the same team therefore a waste of time complaining. No independent body to complain to."

Layers of marginalisation and exclusion, implicit and explicit, serve to delegitimise and silence oppositional voices (Barnes and Bowl, 2001; Barnes and Cotterell, 2012) and thereby block responsiveness.

Caring with

This final phase of care requires that caring needs and the ways in which they are met need to be consistent with democratic commitments to justice, equality and freedom for all. Solidarity.

Tronto's (2013) welcome addition of solidarity by 'caring with' builds on Sevenhuijsen's (1998) acknowledgement of the importance of trust. The ethics of care acknowledges past injustices. Understanding constructions of people who experience madness has a long history. Foucault (1964) discussed the birth of the asylum as a response to how people with mental health problems were removed from prisons as they were thought inferior, Szasz (1960) critiqued psychiatry for a lack of understanding about the 'problems of living' and Goffman (1961) examined the impacts of institutions on the experience of madness. The otherness associated with madness is materialised through the operationalisation of abnormality in psychiatry. Lizzie commented about the denial of human status:

> "The way people get around this is to, in a subtle way, is to deny human status to people that are being treated differently ... We live in a democratic society ... and people haven't got to the point where they are ready to say people with major mental health problems need to be treated just like us ..."

Service users/survivors have called for apologies from the institutions that have treated people with brutality. Josephine had been a 'listener' to people who had been abused in asylums. Participants pondered why change had not occurred despite the considerable efforts of service user/survivor movements, anti-psychiatry movements and recent acknowledgements of social exclusions, stigma and discriminations. Lizzie reflected on the successes of the survivor movement:

> "I think you can, if you look at the women's movement, the gay liberation movement and the Māori renaissance movement and the civil rights movement, they have made more gains than we [survivor movement] have, and that saddens me ... The big issue that got people out in the 1970s was forced treatment and there is more forced treatment going on now, and services have more jurisdiction ... So that, compulsory treatment, has got to be the hot issue – that is the issue that is stopping services developing, it is the boulder in the middle of the road to achieve a recovery orientated service."

Addressing the enduring nature of compulsion would indicate a significant shift in the willingness of services to acknowledge previous harms that service users have encountered, and open a discussion about the possibility of review of the use of compulsion. Solidarity, rather than participation, between services and service users to develop services that meet needs could provide a way of thinking about how to orientate partnerships for real change.

This ethics of care analysis reveals actions that attempted to shut down and minimise the voices of people who experience distress, and a lack of skilled intervention to help people recover. Despite concerted efforts to raise public awareness and challenge discrimination, and to uncover the realities of the mental health system, those who live with mental illness feel that little has changed in terms of the positioning and treatment of people in their situation. With the introduction of community-based compulsion, control has been extended rather than tempered, and rights are not available to people who are compelled to use services. Systematic marginalisation and exclusion are experienced, justified by poorly constructed and heavily critiqued frameworks of illness and over-exaggeration or ill-considered responses to risk. Yet people who are in need require a response, and at times that response may include control. Procedural rights are necessary to ensure proper treatment in the way that control is exercised, but are inadequate for access to redress and cannot address the fundamental injustices experienced by those living with severe mental illness. What is required is care that is guided by Tronto's integrity of care in order to provide protection when it is absolutely required, but that this should be judged with care. Justice requires care.

The integrity of care is potentially transformative as a guide for practice and as a critique of caring practices, as it provides specific critiques of practices between people that achieve or impede the aims of care. It reinstates the dynamics of relationships as central to caring practices between all of the people involved. Each one of the elements of the integrity of care has transformative potential. Attentiveness requires all of the actors involved to state their needs, but services rarely state what their needs are in a given situation, such as the need to maintain a person's safety and therefore limit their freedom. Such a statement of need may well crystallise the intent of services to use force, for example. Responsibility to meet needs would mean that services were unable to justify not meeting needs as a limitation of their service boundary. Competence would mean that the (lack of) necessary resources to provide care was clearly stated, a level of advocacy that most practitioners would welcome. Responsiveness ensures that there is a service user's perspective about care. Finally, solidarity would pave the way for a meaningful renewal of governance and leadership in a partnership between people who provide services and those who use them.

An ethics of care has a central political argument for equality. People who experience mental health problems often do so as a consequence of life events, such as trauma and interpersonal violence, often complicated by poverty, a lack of opportunities and material and social resources. Identifying needs, finding the right responses, with a responsibility to create and sustain change is transformative. Detailed knowledge of lived experiences is necessary to understand what responses are required. This complex, situated knowledge provides direction for responses to alleviate inequality. Everyday experiences are about everyday life and are not restricted to particular services, so it is necessary for a societal responsibility to alleviate inequality, beyond a response that is limited to health and social services.

One societal responsibility is to consider how people who depend on others are valued. Tronto recognises that dependency has long been linked to a pathology of the individual, and therefore whether that person is an (in)adequate citizen (2013, p 150). Health and social services reflect and construct societal norms regarding social worth. In mental health discourses, dependence and independence are embedded in the notions of (lack of) self-reliance and resilience, and close self-surveillance of health behaviours such as adequate sleep, decreasing anxieties and healthy eating. Little or no attention is given to the adversity that people face. Services emphasise decreasing personal risks for service users and encouraging the use of medication for the control of symptoms. Emphasis on risk management and medications obscures what service users actually need from services in order to deal with poverty, unemployment, disrupted education or practical help. Care is broader than clinical services that aim to decrease the symptoms of mental illness. Multiple and varied services are required that respond to the complex and situated lived experiences of service users. In times of austerity and rationalisation, there is a tendency to assume that to receive any service is fortunate, and clinical services are favoured over community services for funding. This creates a situation where many people do not receive the care that they require, and are also faced with services that are coloured by the potential for compulsory action against them. Limiting the options for care by prioritising clinical services may lead to a provision of services that are not experienced as care. Assuming that all care is good may 'allow ourselves to be misled by the ways in which care functions discursively to obscure injustices' (Tronto, 2013, p 24).

Transformations in mental health services

Justice may be understood here to describe the level of acceptance and challenge that occurs within our societies to reform or make change. Tronto (2013) suggests that the ethics of care takes central stage in the articulation of morality and the achievement of care. Justice may be possible by surfacing the morality of the politics of mental health service provision, and the various forms of challenge from survivor movements, antipsychiatry, anti-discriminatory practices and feminism. The ethics of care is a challenge to the current accepted moralities that enable practices that perpetuate injustices. Given the past injustices in psychiatry, equality can be attempted only with recognition of these past injustices. Unless there is a way to articulate these issues, then inequality will continue.

Taking these factors into consideration prompts the question of what kind of caring practices and institutions are required (Tronto, 2010). Service provision is influenced by politics, policy and professional domains of practice. Participants were unequivocal about the role of compulsion, describing it as 'the boulder in the road' that prevented recovery-based services, that added to rather than helped to alleviate distress. This made life unnecessarily much harder than it needed to be. Desirable services, provided by people who understood their experience, had the aims of helping people to enable themselves to decrease their distress. Legislative rights reinforced power and incapacity, when humanness and connection was wanted, along with a sense of hope and practical help that attended to the social problems of poor housing and unemployment that people faced. Removing the focus on abnormality, challenging stigma and discrimination that stops people accessing resources, and providing the sorts of help that would solve social need would go a long way in achieving justice.

EIGHTEEN

Conclusion: renewal and transformation – the importance of an ethics of care

Marian Barnes, Tula Brannelly, Lizzie Ward and Nicki Ward

In the introduction to this collection we highlighted the value of the ethics of care not only in enabling a critique of policy and practice, but as a way of transforming this. Here we offer further reflections drawing on the specific contributions made by chapter authors. The ethics of care is a way of thinking about politics, social practices and the everyday-life considerations of people in diverse circumstances. It provides a perspective that connects values – the things that 'matter' to people (Sayer, 2011), the practical help and support they need when times are hard, the relationships through which they feel recognised and valued and the political priorities that govern public decision making. We write this at a time when confidence in democratic systems is at a low ebb. People are frustrated at the apparent lack of political will to address concerns about inequality, adequate health services, fair and equal rights, decent employment rights and a living wage. Despite the fall-out from the 2008 financial crisis, the supremacy of market values remains largely unquestioned. Enduring inequalities and injustice reach beyond the local and national to the global. Disillusionment with the political establishment's willingness to confront injustice undermines confidence in democracy.

What can the ethics of care contribute in this situation? Care is part of everyone's everyday lives; the issues that care raises about how we live together, what we think is good or 'right', and how we take responsibility for the allocation of resources to meet basic human needs are enduring ones. Care is political. Questions about who cares for whom have long been recognised by feminists as political as well as personal issues. As demographic shifts and global mobility foreground questions of who cares for an ageing population, we confront the dangers of intergenerational conflict. This conflict, and the broader debates about 'fairness' and 'deservedness' in relation to welfare, are constructed within 'common sense' neoliberal assumptions about the limits within which public spending should be focused on ensuring well-being (Hall and O'Shea, 2013). While politicians appeal to 'hard working families' as the bedrock of society, Tronto (2013) asks how society can be organised to acknowledge and prioritise the caring relationships and responsibilities that people, often women, have in their lives, in a balance with work responsibilities. Reflecting on the way families in diverse situations try to determine the 'best' thing to do in order to ensure care for each other, Williams (2004a) emphasises the necessity of balancing the work ethic with the care ethic because people feel pressured to exercise responsibilities to undertake paid work and have little time to care. Williams's work, and that of many other commentators, highlights the way in which values associated with contributions through participating in the labour market are seen to trump those associated with care within the 'private sphere'.

One of our aims in this collection has been to highlight care ethics' insistence on the necessity of knowledge generated from lived experiences of care practices as a basis on which to realise the transformative potential of care thinking. A second, linked aim has been to reassert the necessity of the critical, political character of the feminist ethics of care. Writing in the late 1990s, Hekman (1999) suggested that the feminist movement needed a new 'theory and method' in order to consider the future of difference. She was dismissive of feminist care ethics, suggesting that this reinforced hegemonic Western traditions; what was needed, she suggested, was 'an epistemological alternative that provides an understanding of multiple moral voices' (Hekman, 1999, p 94). We argue that developments in feminist ethics of care do provide such a theory and method. Within this text we have seen the ethics of care applied to a range of geographic and cultural contexts and experiences; to new and emerging phenomena; to an understanding of moral agency expressed in different voices, in critical analyses of current policy discourse, and in making visible the ethical dilemmas associated with professional practices. In so doing, contributors demonstrate its resonance as a theoretical and methodological framework for understanding and exploring the world as well as for providing a language in which care practices can be negotiated. Contributions confirm the significance of the broad definition of care offered by Fisher and Tronto (1990). But challenges remain and we need to name these.

Barriers, challenges and opportunities

Achieving change requires understanding what gets in the way of this. There are many barriers, both for individuals and in terms of the broader political project embodied in feminist care ethics. The broad-based and multi-disciplinary nature of work in this field is both a strength and a weakness. Care ethics can be broadly understood as encompassing many different positions within historical and temporal contexts. In framing this book we aimed to highlight the transformative potential of feminist care ethics as a distinctly *political* project. For example, by foregrounding the centrality of care it is possible, as Anke Niehof (Chapter Eleven) argues, to confer authority on women's decisions, skills and work in ways that can unsettle patriarchy. The global reach of arguments about the centrality of care (Tronto, Chapter Three), and the resonance with indigenous knowledge systems that offer counter-arguments to dominant assumptions about development (Boulton and Brannelly, Chapter Six) demonstrate the aim of the feminist ethics of care to challenge and transform in both theory and practice. This position is distinct from perspectives that combine a focus on care with ideas drawn from 'maternal' feminism or virtue ethics and that divorce care from its political significance. Claiming the significance of care in diverse contexts means that we need to understand the complexity of relational, social and temporal conceptions of care if we are to advance care ethics as a transformative practice (Barnes, Chapter Three).

The apparent similarities between the ethics of care and communitarianism have been critically examined (Kittay, 2001a). Neither developing individual virtues of compassion, nor arguing for collective responsibility without recognising the impact of structural disadvantage and the profoundly oppressive nature of unequal social relations, can deliver the transformative objectives of feminist care ethics. Without an explicitly political stance, arguments for prioritising care can be safely taken on board within the existing power structures and comfortably accommodated in regressive political agendas. As Lizzie Ward (Chapter Four) has argued, care can be invoked within very different discourses: active citizenship, volunteering, promoting active communities and self-care may sound like good things (and even are when they are spontaneously organised collectively through solidarity and common cause), but have vastly different meanings when framed within an agenda committed to actively dismantling public/collective infrastructure for welfare and health. Part of feminist care ethics as a political project must be the on-going and continuous questioning of the ways in which the language and ideas about care are mobilised, and in support of whose interests.

Central to a political ethic of care is the question of *responsibility* (Tronto, 2013). Tronto's conceptualisation of responsibility is relational, as the relationship provides opportunities for responsibility. Taking responsibility involves making change and so is action orientated. Responsibility is not an obligation or duty as in a rights-based understanding, and is not concerned with apportioning blame or praise, and therefore differs from virtue ethics. It is forward looking, relational, negotiated and dynamic, consistent with Margaret Walker's (2007) conceptualisation of the ethic of responsibility. As responsibility is about action, it allows us to move beyond critique and resistance, to renewal and change.

Relationships most frequently involve people in need, and people who meet those needs through direct care giving. As this mainly happens within family and friend relationships, or by paid care givers, relationships between people of privilege and care receivers remain rare. These conditions maintain a situation of continuing privileged irresponsibility (Tronto, 1993, p 120) where those who benefit most from the way care is structured are the last to recognise its importance and influence or to understand the conditions of life for people where needs are unmet.

Identification and analysis of privileged irresponsibility is key to the project of renewal. Privilege resides where people feel at home in the world, and where their needs are met through social, political, economic and other resources (Bozalek, 2011, and Chapter Seven). Marginalisation exists where people are excluded from access to these resources and where needs for care are considered a marker of low value. Irresponsibility marks where people accept their own privilege but not their responsibility for the lack of attention to and resources available to others. Surfacing privilege and how it operates is one aspect of identification, and connects personal lives with political contexts. Bozalek's (Chapter Seven) work in social work education illustrates the value of enabling future practitioners to develop attentiveness through reflecting on care within their own lives.

The personal *is* political

Fundamental to the processes of change is the embodiment of personal, professional and political insights. It is notable that a number of scholars working in this tradition incorporate personal narratives (their own or drawn from the experiences of others) in building their arguments. For example, Eva Kittay, a moral philosopher, draws heavily from her personal experience as the mother of a disabled daughter to develop her conceptions of care and justice. At the level of face-to-face care she illustrates the value of what we might understand as a 'dialogic process without words' when she reflects on how her daughter contributed to the practice of care without being able to speak the words for this (Kittay, 1999, p 157). And at the level of philosophical analysis she castigates her colleagues who are not prepared to engage with lived experience of cognitive disability before drawing conclusions about the moral worth of disabled people (Kittay, 2010). As a philosopher, Kittay is troubled by her departure from the norms that govern the practice of her discipline when she draws on personal experience to challenge professional colleagues. It is worth quoting her self-questioning at some length – she is reflecting after a conference where she had made such a challenge:

> What, I wondered, was I doing in a discipline that thought it appropriate to question the full worth of a portion of humanity, one that happened to include my daughter? A discipline whose practitioners sat on the sidelines as I fought to defend her moral worth and that of those like her?
>
> … This chapter … is a meditation on the conversation that closed the conference, and it is a reflection on my dual role: philosopher, and also stakeholder in the philosophical debate – though not just any stakeholder, but a mother. Can one do good philosophy, be practically efficacious, and keep intact the relationship of mother and child, or are the difficulties in this project insurmountable? Are there philosophical and practical payoffs in making philosophy this personal – and do they justify the personal costs of the effort? (Kittay, 2010, p 395)

All of us (editors) have found ourselves drawing on and reflecting on personal experience as we develop our professional and political projects of working with the ethics of care. And when we have introduced this perspective (in the context of research and teaching) to others who might be identified as both care givers and care receivers we have experienced positive responses, sometimes including relief, at finding a framework within which to make sense of and explore dilemmas and tensions. Responses to the ethics of care include a sense of urgency and rationale to give credence to positions that people find are heavily challenged in their work. For example Liveng (Chapter Ten) demonstrates the discomfort that many practitioners feel when policy discourse does not reflect the reality of day-to-day practice. Taking this a stage further would enable the renewal offered by care ethics through its empirical as well as ethical focus.

A number of contributors to this collection demonstrate the value of working with personal experience to offer reimaginings of care. Both Ann Fudge Schormans (Chapter Fourteen) and Nicki Ward (Chapter Thirteen) draw from research with people with learning disabilities to contribute insights that unsettle the care giver/care receiver dichotomy and, in doing so, also illuminate the value of care ethics in understanding power relations in care. The background to negotiations about including the images that are the focus of the analysis recorded by Fudge Schormans offers another perspective on power and also demonstrates the limitations of a justice perspective. 'Ownership' of these images rests with the photographer through copyright law. As the originator of the images, this person has the right to control their use, regardless of the impact they may have on those depicted and without a responsibility to enable public dialogue about this. Those whose lives are subject to others' gaze can find it hard to make a public challenge to the constructions those images reinforce. In a rather different context from that explored by Niehof (Chapter Eleven), these contributions suggest how expertise in care has the potential to confer value on those too often devalued, but achieving this remains a struggle. Bozalek (Chapter Seven) discusses how transformation may be achieved through encouraging personal reflections among black, working-class South African social work students. Diego de Merich (Chapter Eight) also considers the transformative impact of a project that encourages personal reflections among fathers in relation to experiences of parenting. And Evans and Atim (Chapter Twelve) illustrate the significance of the emotional dimensions of care in the stories they recount of young people involved in the care of family members with AIDS/HIV.

Renewing care through dialogue

What unites these very different contributions is something that those interested in the practical implications of care ethics have long highlighted – that this necessitates a dialogic and narrative form of practice (for example Parton, 2003). And this, in turn, emphasises the epistemic significance of the part played by the care receiver in the care process. The locations in which such practices take place are not only those in which personal care is given and received, but also those in which policy decisions are debated and knowledge about care is generated.

Marian Barnes (2008) has argued that, to Tronto and Sevenhuijsen's emphasis on the necessity of deliberating *about* care as a core dimension of policy and politics, we need to add the importance of deliberating *with* care. She argues that Tronto's dimensions of care – attentiveness, responsibility, competence and responsiveness – can be applied to the process of deliberation involving those usually seen as care receivers, as well as to what is more usually thought of as care. As Kittay's experience demonstrates, including lived experience within the debate will frequently question not only the topic of deliberation but also the way in which deliberation is conducted, and that is the case whether that be in the context of an academic discipline or the policy process (Barnes, 2002, 2008). Walker (2007) bases her arguments for feminist ethics within a similar recognition of the need to practise philosophy differently in order to reach different conclusions. In the world of practical social policy there are many experiences of failed 'involvement' initiatives that demonstrate that simply putting public officials and older people, people with mental health problems or others who may be defined as users of services together in a room does not lead to either understanding or real change in policy or practice. And both empirical and theoretical work on deliberative democracy suggests that what gets in the way of change is often an unwillingness to recognise and give credence to ways of speaking outside institutional norms, as well as an unwillingness to control and define legitimate knowledge in these contexts (Barnes, Newman and Sullivan, 2007). Adapting a quotation from Tronto about care, Barnes has suggested: 'Intending to enable people to take part in policy making, even taking responsibility to set up opportunities for this to happen, but then failing to conduct deliberation in a way that enables people to feel their contributions are recognised and valued, means that the purpose of participation is not fulfilled' (Barnes, 2012a, p 162).

In Canada Kathryn Church's (1996) study of involving mental health service users provided a clear example of how public officials continued to distance themselves from service users whom they had invited to take part – in this instance by constructing the expression of pain and anger in the context of discussions about service design as evidence of 'bad manners' in the process of debate. As Brannelly (Chapter Seventeen) demonstrates, mental health service users continue to experience othering that undermines potentially positive experiences of care and that amounts to injustice. The value of working with both the ethics of care and theories of intersectionality (Ward, Chapter Five) is that it can sensitise us to ways in which different identities are constituted through processes of giving and receiving care, and within those contexts in which policies and practices for care are being deliberated. These contributions offer important insights into both the necessity of care for social justice and the value of care thinking, together with a commitment to participatory decision making within welfare policies and services.

Interpersonal relations, subjectivity and identity

One aspect of the power of the ethics of care is its capacity to make sense to 'ordinary people' as a way of reflecting on the significance of care and caring relations in their lives. It also offers some different perspectives that challenge dominant assumptions about the relevance and meaning of care in everyday lives. Ward and Fudge Schormans have considered this with respect to those traditionally recognised as 'care receivers', but Manea (Chapter Sixteen) also invites us to recognise the importance of care for those who might be considered to occupy the kind of powerful positions that obscure vulnerabilities. If real transformation is to be achieved, then it is necessary for those who deny their need for care to recognise this.

It may be easier in the context of work with older people for practitioners to move away from the 'them and us' positioning that distances some practitioners from recognising that care is something we all need, because, although many people resist ageing and seek to distance themselves from their own older self, ageing is more likely to be recognised as something we will all/most experience than is mental illness, for example. Is this something that might encourage a wider recognition of the importance of care as more are involved in care of ageing parents and start to acknowledge their own ageing? Can such awareness start to change the way in which we think about the significance of care more widely? While this may be the case, and the renewal of care may well be helped by demographic changes and personal experiences resulting from this, we suggest that there is also a need for positive action to encompass ways of working based on the ethics of care in diverse processes of democratic policy making, including research to influence policy (Ward and Gahagan, 2010).

Practising care

We have suggested that renewal or transformation can and should take place in different spaces and we have considered this in the context of politics and discourse, in relation to policy and policy making and in relation to subjectivities and interpersonal relationships. Our contributors also explore the significance of care ethics in relation to renewing caring practices.

In Chapter Nine Moser and Thygesen dispute the assumption that care is replaced by technology and instead highlight how care networks can embrace technology and the new practices this can enable. But for this to happen in a way that can improve the lives of care givers and receivers, the value of care must be asserted rather than denied. Liveng (Chapter Ten) focuses on the frustrations and discomforts of those practitioners asked to adopt ways of thinking and working that do not reflect their recognition of the value of communication, interaction and relationships with service users. Steckley (Chapter Fifteen) reveals the unfamiliarity of ethical concepts to many practitioners, while suggesting that such ideas may be at least implicit in the way they negotiate the right thing to do in difficult contexts. All these contributions suggest that an explicit adoption of a care ethics language and perspective could provide a starting point for a dialogue about what constitutes good care, and that this would benefit both those working at care and those who are dependent on care. As we have suggested, the ethics of care draws attention to specific contexts and highlights the need for dialogue between those involved in care relationships in order to determine the best action in the specific situation. Care networks (Barnes, Chapter Three) may involve practitioners from different disciplines. Because the ethics of care is not a professional ethics based in specific practices it has the potential to facilitate interprofessional dialogue, as well as dialogue between professionals and service users (Barnes and Brannelly, 2008; Banks, 2010). A language that enables such conversations increases the potential for the transformation of caring relationships.

Solidarity and social justice

The face-to-face, everyday experience of giving and receiving care is often the starting point for understanding injustices experienced by those in need of care. In her article 'Creating Caring Institutions', Tronto (2010) argues that care is 'purposive'. If this is the case, then we need to ask what purpose care should achieve. Adding 'caring with' to the four phases of care, Tronto (2013) names the importance of solidarity as part of care thinking. Our political perspective on care ethics is one that assumes that thinking care and justice together is fundamental and that achieving justice requires care (Kittay, 1999). While we need to distinguish care ethics from justice ethics this is because we need to understand how both are necessary to social justice, rather than in order to decide which position to adopt.

Although poor (and sometimes abusive) experiences of using services undermine any sense of being cared for, many practitioners recognise and struggle with how their practices can link to the social justice values they hold. 'Abandoning' care (Barnes, 2011) in favour of choice and control is unlikely to be the answer. The distinction of 'doing with' rather than 'doing to' when working with vulnerable populations repositions and strengthens the need for resources in order to care well.

Making a link between micro-level interactions and the processes of collective decision making is one means through which the personal and the political can connect. This requires participative policy processes that enable explicit and public dialogue about the relationship between care and justice. Theoretically, there are useful contributions from beyond ethics–of–care scholarship that point to the nature of such connections: Nancy Fraser's (1997, 2009) work on transformative recognition and on participatory parity as necessary components of social justice and Iris Marion Young's (2011) social connection model of justice. Both suggest that understanding justice in terms of competing rights is not the most helpful basis on which to achieve change. A relational perspective points to the inadequacy of an approach, for example, that suggests that either service users' or lay carers' rights should be prioritised. Not only does this fail to attend to the relationship between them, but it essentialises the dichotomous identities of care giver and receiver. As Ward (Chapter Five) has shown, care ethics resonates with work that explores the way that the intersectional experiences of identity are constructed.

In the applied contexts that are the main foci of our work and of many contributions to this collection we see real benefits in promoting a dialogue about the necessity of care to justice. This can be a means of addressing critiques of care from within the disability movement, but also avoiding a consequent apparent alliance between disability activism and the marketisation of welfare. Some disability activists – Jenny Morris, Tom Shakespeare – have recognised the potential of such a dialogue (Morris, 2001; Shakespeare, 2006). Within this collection Boulton and Brannelly (Chapter Six) think together care and justice through a consideration of Māori values and the experiences of colonised, indigenous peoples. Ruth Evans and Agnes Atim (Chapter Twelve) link the participation of people living with AIDS/HIV in Tanzania and Uganda to improved access to healthcare, while Joan Tronto (Chapter Two) reflects on care and justice at a global level. This perspective also reminds us that many of those who work at care are themselves in vulnerable positions as workers (Boccagni, 2014) and that the interests of both workers and service users may be better served in campaigning *for* rather than *against* care.

Conclusion

The previous points demonstrate that we do not propose care ethics alone as the theoretical or political 'solution' to the personal and political challenges associated with care. Care ethics does not provide all the answers but it does, we argue, enable questions to be asked and a framework to be applied not only for critical analysis, but to suggest ways forward to renew care, justice and subjective experience. The power of the ethics of care lies in its capacity to move between the messy everyday realities of care giving and receiving, and the political processes through which policy is made, while applying a coherent philosophical and psychological understanding of interdependence as fundamental to the human condition.

References

Adewunmi, B. (2014) 'Kimberlé Crenshaw on intersectionality: "I wanted to come up with an everyday metaphor that anyone could use"', *New Statesman*, 2 April, www.newstatesman.com/lifestyle/2014/04/kimberl-crenshaw-intersectionality-i-wanted-come-everyday-metaphor-anyone-could (accessed 23 July 2014).

Agosta, L. (1984) 'Empathy and Intersubjectivity', in J. Lichtenberg, M. Bornstein and D. Silver (eds) *Empathy I*, Hillsdale, NJ: The Analytic Press, pp 43–61.

Agosta, L. (2010) *Empathy in the Context of Philosophy*, Basingstoke: Palgrave Macmillan.

Akintola, O. (2006) 'Gendered home-based care in South Africa: more trouble for the troubled', *African Journal of AIDS Research*, vol 5, no 3, pp 237–47.

Allen, D. (2008) 'Risk and prone restraint: reviewing the evidence', in M.A. Nunno, D.M. Day, and L.B. Bullard (eds) *For Our Own Safety: Examining the Safety of High-risk Interventions for Children and Young People*, Arlington, VA: Child Welfare League of America, Inc, pp 87–106.

Allen, D. (2013) 'A connected society', *Soundings*, no 53, pp 103–13.

Allen, P. and Sachs, C. (2012) 'Women and food chains; the gendered politics of food', in P. Williams-Forson and C. Counihan (eds) *Taking Food Public: Redefining Foodways in a Changing World*, New York and London: Routledge, pp 23–40.

Ally, S. (2009) *From Servants to Workers: South African Domestic Workers and the Democratic State*, New York: Cornell University Press.

Anglin, J.P. (2002) *Pain, Normality, and the Struggle for Congruence: Reinterpreting Residential Child Care for Children and Youth*, New York: The Haworth Press.

Anthias, F. (2013) 'Intersectional what? Social divisions, intersectionality and levels of analysis', *Ethnicities*, vol 13, no 1, pp 3–19.

Arnfred, S. (2007) 'Sex, food and female power: Discussion of data material from Northern Mozambique', *Sexualities*, vol 10, no 2, pp 141–58.

Aronson, J. and Smith, K. (2010) 'Managing restructured social services: Expanding the social?', *British Journal of Social Work*, vol 40, pp 530–47.

Aronson, J. and Smith, K. (2011) 'Identity work and critical social services management: Balancing on a tightrope?', *British Journal of Social Work*, vol 41, pp 432–48.

Asante, M.K. (1988) *Afrocentricity*, Trenton, NJ: Africa World Press.

Ash, A. (2010) 'Ethics and the street-level bureaucrat: Implementing policy to protect elders from abuse', *Ethics and Social Welfare*, vol 4, pp 201–9.

Asia Pulse Staff (2009) 'Sri Lanka doctors, accountants lead brain drain: study', *Asia Pulse*, Colombo.

Audit Commission (1993) *Performance review in local government: A handbook for auditors and local authorities*, London: Audit Commission.

Baggini, J. (2012) 'Why politicians are making morality fashionable again', *Guardian*, 24 July www.guardian.co.uk/world/2012/jul/24/why-morality-is-fashionable-again?INTCMP=SRCH (accessed 28 July 2012).

Bailey, A. (2000) 'Locating traitorous identities: toward a view of privilege-cognisant white character', in U. Narayan and S. Harding (eds) *Decentring The Center. Philosophy for a Multicultural, Postcolonial, and Feminist World*, Bloomington and Indianapolis: Indiana University Press.

Baker, C., Johnson, K., Virgo, L. and Ward, N. (2012) 'Fulfilling potential consultation: The views of people with learning disabilities who are carers', unpublished report, www.birmingham.ac.uk/Documents/college-social-sciences/social-policy/IASS/research/fulfilling-potential-consultation.pdf.

Banks, S. (2010) 'Interprofessional ethics: a developing field? Notes from the *Ethics and Social Welfare* Conference, Sheffield UK, May 2010', *Ethics and Social Welfare*, vol 4, no 3, pp 280–94.

Baputaki, C. (2009) 'Botswana; Nursing is Plagued By "Brain Drain"', *Africa News*, 26 June.

Bargh, M. (2007) *Resistance: An Indigenous Response to Neoliberalism*, Wellington: Huia Publishers.

Barnes, M. (2002) 'Bringing difference into deliberation. Disabled people, survivors and local governance' *Policy & Politics*, vol 30, no 3, pp 355–68.

Barnes, M. (2006) *Caring and Social Justice*, Basingstoke: Palgrave MacMillan.

Barnes, M. (2007) 'Participation, citizenship and a feminist ethic of care', in S. Balloch and M. Hill (eds) *Communities, Citizenship and Care: Research and Practice in a Changing Policy Context*, Bristol: Policy Press, pp 59–74.

Barnes, M. (2008) 'Passionate participation: emotional experiences and expressions in deliberative forums', *Critical Social Policy*, vol 28, no 4, pp 461–81.

Barnes, M. (2011) 'Abandoning care? a critical perspective on personalisation from an ethic of care', *Ethics and Social Welfare*, vol 5, no 2, pp 153–67.

Barnes, M. (2011b) 'Caring responsibilities. The making of citizen carers', in J. Newman and E. Tonkens (eds) *Participation, Responsibility and Choice: Summoning the Active Citizen in Western European Welfare States*, Amsterdam: University of Amsterdam Press, pp 161-78.

Barnes, M. (2012a) *Care in Everyday Life: An ethic of care in practice*, Bristol: Policy Press.

Barnes, M. (2012b) 'An ethic of care and sibling care in older age', *Families, Relationships and Societies*, vol 1, no 1, pp 7–24.

Barnes, M. and Bowl, R. (2001) *Taking over the Asylum*, Basingstoke: Palgrave.

Barnes, M. and Brannelly, T. (2008) 'Achieving care and social justice for people with dementia', *Nursing Ethics*, vol 15, pp 384–95.

Barnes, M. and Cotterell, P. (eds) (2012) *Critical Perspectives on User Involvement*, Bristol: Policy Press.

Barnes, M. and Henwood, F. (2015) 'Inform with care: Ethics and information in care for people with dementia', *Ethics and Social Welfare*, vol 9, no 2, pp 147–63.

Barnes, M., Henwood, F. and Smith, N. (2014) 'Information and care: a relational approach', *Dementia,* DOI 10.1177/1471301214527750.

Barnes, M., Newman, J. and H. Sullivan (2007) *Power, Participation and Political Renewal: Case studies in public participation*, Bristol: Policy Press.

Barnett, T. (2006) 'HIV/AIDS, nutrition and food security: Looking to future challenges', in S. Gillespie (ed) *AIDS, Poverty and Hunger: Challenges and Responses*, Washington DC: IFPRI, pp 341–49.

Baron-Cohen, S. (2011) *Zero Degrees of Empathy: A New Theory of Human Cruelty*, London: Allen Lane Books.

Bauman, Z. (2006) *Liquid Fear*, Cambridge: Polity Press.

BBC (2013a) 'David Cameron defiant over tougher EU benefit plans', 27 November, www.bbc.co.uk/news/uk-politics-25114890 (accessed 22 June 2015).

BBC (2013b) 'Councils prepare for migrant influx of Bulgarians and Romanians', 3 December, www.bbc.co.uk/news/uk-25206972 (accessed 22 June 2015).

BBC (2013c) 'Migration pressure fears for school places', 3 December, www.bbc.co.uk/news/uk-england-25207124 (accessed 22 June 2015).

Beaumont, J. and Cloke, P. (eds) (2012) *Faith-based Organisations and Exclusion in European Cties*, Bristol: Policy Press.

Beckett, C. (2007) 'Women, disability, care: Good neighbours or uneasy bedfellows?', *Critical Social Policy*, vol 27, no 3, pp 360–80.

Beckmann, N. and Bujra, J. (2010) 'The politics of the queue: The politicization of People living with HIV/AIDS in Tanzania', *Development and Change*, vol 41, no 6, pp 1041–64.

Bell, D.A. (2001) 'Equal Rights for Foreign Resident Workers?', *Dissent*, vol 48, pp 26–34.

Bella, L. (2010) 'In sickness and in health: public and private responsibility for health care from Bismarck to Obama', in R. Harris, C.N. Wathen and S. Wyatt (eds) *Configuring Health Consumers: Health work and the imperative of personal responsibility*, Basingstoke: Palgrave Macmillan, pp 13–29.

Beneréria, L. (2008) 'The crisis of care, international migration, and public policy', *Feminist Economics*, vol 14, pp 1–21.

Berger, J. and Mohr, J. (2010) *A Seventh Man*, 1st edn 1975, London: Verso.

Bidois, E. (2011) 'A cultural and personal perspective of psychosis', in J. Geekei, P. Randall, J. Read and D. Lampshire (eds) *Experiencing Psychosis: Personal and professional perspectives*, Hove: Routledge.

Boccagni, P. (2014) 'Caring about migrant care workers: from private obligations to transnational social welfare?', *Critical Social Policy*, vol 34, no 2, pp 221–40.

Boler, M. and Zembylas, M. (2003) 'Discomforting truths: The emotional terrain of understanding difference', in P. Trifonas (ed) *Pedagogies of Difference: Rethinking education for social change*, New York: Routledge Falmer, pp 110–36.

Bondi, L. (2008) 'On the relational dynamics of caring: a psychotherapeutic approach to emotional and power dimensions of women's care work', *Gender, Place and Culture*, vol 15, no 3, pp 249–65.

Booth, T. and Booth, W. (2005) 'Parents with learning difficulties in the child protection system: Experiences and perspectives', *Journal of Intellectual Disabilities*, vol 9, no 2, pp 109–29.

Borell, B.A.E., Gregory, A.S., McCreanor, T.N., Jensen, V.G.L. and Moewaka Barnes, H.E. (2009) 'It's hard at the top but it's a whole lot easier than being at the bottom: The Role of Privilege in Understanding Disparities in Aotearoa–New Zealand', *Race/Ethnicity*, vol 3, no 1, pp 29–50.

Boris, E. and Parreñas, R.S. (2010) *Intimate Labors: Cultures, Technologies, and the Politics of Care*, Stanford, CA: Stanford Social Sciences.

Boulton, A. (2007) 'Taking account of culture: the contracting experience of Māori mental health providers', *AlterNative*, no 3, pp 124–41.

Bowden, P. (2000) 'An "ethic of care", in clinical settings: encompassing "feminine" and "feminist" perspectives', *Nursing Philosophy*, vol 1, no 1, pp 36–49.

Bozalek, V. (2010) 'The effect of institutional racism on student family circumstances: A human capabilities perspective', *South African Journal of Psychology*, vol 40, no 4, pp 487–94.

Bozalek, V. (2011) 'Acknowledging privilege through encounters with difference: Participatory Learning and Action techniques for decolonizing methodologies in Southern contexts', *International Journal of Social Research Methodology*, vol 14, no 6, pp 469–84.

Bozalek, V. (2012) 'Recognition and participatory parity: Students' accounts of gendered family practices', *The Social Work Practitioner-Researcher*, vol 24, no 1, pp 66–84.

Bozalek, V. (2014) 'Privileged irresponsibility', in G. Olthuis, H. Kohlen and J. Heier, J.(eds) *Moral boundaries redrawn: The significance of Joan Tronto's argument for political theory, professional ethics and care as a practice*, Leuven: Peeters.

Bozalek, V., Carolissen, R. and Leibowitz, B. (2014) 'A pedagogy of hope in South African Higher Education', in V. Bozalek, B. Leibowitz, R. Carolissen and M. Boler (eds) *Discerning Critical Hope in Educational Practices*, London and New York: Routledge.

Brannelly, P.M. (2006) 'Negotiating ethics in dementia care. An analysis of an ethic of care in practice', *Dementia*, vol 5, no 2, pp 197–212.

Brannelly, T. (2010) 'Sustaining citizenship: People with dementia and the phenomenon of social death', *Nursing Ethics*, vol 18, no 5, pp 662–71.

Brannelly, T. (2011) 'That others matter the moral achievement – care ethics and citizenship in practice with people with dementia', *Ethics and Social Welfare*, vol 5, no 2, pp 210–16.

Brannelly, T., Boulton, A. and Te Hiini, A. (2013) 'A relationship between the ethics of care and Māori worldview – the place of relationality and care in Māori mental health service provision', *Ethics and Social Welfare*, vol 7, no 4, pp 410–22. DOI 10.1080/17496535.2013.764001.

Buchan, J. (2001) 'Nurses moving across borders: "brain drain"or freedom of movement?', *International Nursing Review*, vol 48, pp 65.

Budlender, D. (2010a) 'Tanzania: Care in the context of HIV and AIDS', in D. Budlender (ed) *Time Use Studies and Unpaid Care Work*, New York and London: Routledge, pp 46–68.

Budlender, D. (2010b) 'South Africa: When marriage and the nuclear family are not the norm', in D. Budlender (ed) *Time Use Studies and Unpaid Care Work*, New York and London: Routledge, pp 69–91.

Busfield, J. (2010) 'A pill for every ill: Explaining the expansion in medicine use', *Social Science and Medicine*, vol 70, pp 934–41.

Butler, J. (2004) *Precarious Life: The powers of mourning and violence*, London: Verso.

Cangiano, A., Shutes, I. et al (2009) *Migrant Care Workers in Ageing Societies: Research Findings in the United Kingdom*, Oxford: Compas.

Card, C. (1995) *Lesbian Choices*, New York: Columbia University Press.

Carers Trust (2014) 'Taking care of yourself', www.carers.org/help-directory/taking-care-yourself (accessed 27 February 2014).

Carers UK (2014) 'Looking After Yourself', www.carersuk.org/help-and-advice/looking-after-you, (accessed 27th February 2014).

Carnaby, S. and Cambridge, P. (2006) *Intimate and Personal Care with People with Learning Disabilities*, London: Jessica Kingsley.

Cataldo, F., Museheke, M. and Kielmann, K. (2008) 'New challenges for home-based care providers in the context of ARTroll-out in Zambia', XVII International AIDS Conference, Mexico City, 2–8 August, abstract number MOPE0167.

Cehan, I. and Manea, T. (2012) 'International codes of medical recruitment: evolution and efficiency', *Romanian Journal of Bioethics*, vol 10, no 1, pp 100–9.

Chambers, R. (1981) 'Editorial introduction: vulnerability, coping and policy', *IDS Bulletin*, vol 20, no 2, pp 1–7.

Chambers, R. (2005) *Ideas for Development*, London: Earthscan.

Champagne, T. and Stromberg, N. (2004) 'Sensory approaches in inpatient psychiatric settings: Innovative alternatives to seclusion and restraint', *Journal of Psychosocial Nursing and Mental Health Services*, vol 42, pp 34–44.

Chattoo, S. and Ahmad, W.I.U. (2008) 'The moral economy of selfhood and caring: negotiating boundaries of personal care as embodied moral practice', *Sociology of Health and Illness*, vol 30, no 4, pp 550–64.

Chimwaza, A. and Watkins, S. (2004) 'Giving care to people with symptoms of AIDS in rural sub-Saharan Africa', *AIDS Care*, vol 16, no 7, pp 795–807.

Church, K. (1996) 'Beyond "bad manners": the power relations of "consumer participation", in Ontario's Community Mental Health System', *Canadian Journal of Community Mental Health*, vol 15, no 2, pp 22–5.

Clacherty, G. and Donald, D. (2006) *Impact Evaluation of the VSI (Vijana Simama Imara) Organisation and the Rafiki Mdogo Group of the HUMULIZA Orphan Project, Nshamba, Tanzania*, Johannesburg: Novartis Foundation for Sustainable Development and Regional Psychosocial Support Initiative.

Clarke, J. (2005) 'New Labour's citizens: activated, empowered, responsibilized, abandoned?', *Critical Social Policy*, vol 25, no 4, pp 447–63.

Clark Miller, S. (2010) 'Cosmopolitan care', *Ethics and Social Welfare*, vol 4, no 2, pp 145–57.

Cock, J. (1989) *Maids and Madams: Domestic Workers Under Apartheid*, London: The Women's Press.

Colton, D. (2004) *Checklist for Assessing your Organization's Readiness for Reducing Seclusion and Restraint*, Staunton, VA: Commonwealth Center for Children and Adolescence, http://rccp.cornell.edu/pdfs/SR%20Checklist%201-Colton.pdf.

Connell, R. (2012) 'Gender, health and theory: Conceptualizing the issue, in local and world perspective', *Social Science & Medicine*, vol 74, pp 1675–83.

Corby, B., Doig, A. and Roberts, V. (2001) *Public Inquiries into Abuse of Children in Residential Care*, London: Jessica Kingsley Publishers.

Cornwall, J. (2006) 'Might is right? A discussion of ethics and practicalities of control and restraint in schools', *Emotional and Behavioural Difficulties*, vol 5, pp 19–25.

Craig, T.J. (2008) 'Major psychiatric disorders increase risk of mortality', *Evidence Based Mental Health*, vol 11, no 9, DOI 10.1136/ebmh.11.1.9.

Crenshaw, K. (1991) 'Mapping the margins: intersectionality, identity politics, and violence against women of color', *Stanford Law Review*, vol 43, no 6, pp 1241–99.

Crittenden, C. (2001) 'The principles of care', *Women and Politics*, vol 22, pp 81–105.

Crozier, G.K.D. (2010) 'Care workers in the global market: appraising application of feminist care ethics', *International Journal of Feminist Approaches to Bioethics*, vol 3, pp 113–37.

Dahl, H.M. (2011) 'Who can be against quality?', in M.E. Purkis et al (eds) *Perspectives on Care at Home for Older People*, London and New York: Routledge, pp 139–57.

Dahlberg, G. and Moss, P. (2005) *Ethics and Politics in Early Childhood Education*, London: Routledge/Falmer.

Darmon, I. and Perez, C. (2011) '"Conduct of conduct" or the shaping of "adequate dispositions"? Labour market and career guidance in four European countries', *Critical Social Policy*, vol 31, no 1, pp 77–101.

Davidson, J. and Milligan, C. (2004) 'Embodying emotion sensing space: introducing emotional geographies', *Social and Cultural Geography*, vol 5, no 4, pp 523–32.

Davidson, J., Mccullough, D., Steckley, L. and Warren, T. (2005) *Holding Safely: A Guide for Residential Child Care Practitioners and Managers about Physically Restraining Children and Young People*, Glasgow: Scottish Institute of Residential Child Care.

Davies, C. and Malik, S. (2014) 'Welcome to Luton: Romanian arrival greeted by two MPs and a media scrum', *Guardian*, 1 January, www.theguardian.com/uk-news/2014/jan/01/luton-romanian-arrival-mps-media (accessed 1 January 2014).

Davies, C.A. (1999) *Reflexive Ethnography. A guide to researching selves and others*, Routledge: London and New York.

Davies, W. (2012) 'The emerging neocommunitarianism', *The Political Quarterly*, vol 83, no 4, pp 767–76.

Day, D.M. (2000) *A Review of the Literature on Restraints and Seclusion with Children and Youth: Toward the development of a perpective in practice. Report to the Intersectoral/Interministerial Steering Committee on Behaviour Management Interventions for Children and Youth in Residential and Hospital Settings*, Toronto, Ontario: The Intersectional/ Interministerial Steering Committee on Behaviour Management Intervention for Children and Youth in Residential and Hospital Settings.

De Beauvoir, S. (1972) *The Second Sex,* Harmondsworth: Penguin.

DH (Department of Health) (2001a) *The National Framework for Older People*, London: Department of Health.

Department of Health (2001b) *Valuing People, A. New Strategy for Learning Disability for the 21st Century,* Cm 5086, London: Department of Health.

Department of Health (2002) 'Requirements for Social Work Training', http://cdn.basw.co.uk/upload/basw_40833-3.pdf.

DH (2005a) *Self Care – A Real Choice*, London: Department of Health.

DH (2005b) *Self Care Support: A compendium of practical examples across the whole system of health and social care*, http://webarchive.nationalarchives. gov.uk/20050202182438/http://dh.gov.uk/prod_consum_dh/ idcplg?IdcService=GET_FILE&dID=620&Rendition=Web (accessed 14 November 2013).

DH (2005c) *Independence Well-Being and Choice: Our Vision for the Future of Adult Social Care in England*, London: Department of Health.

DH (2006) *Our Health, Our Care, Our Say*, London: Department of Health.

DH (2009) *Valuing People Now*, London: Department of Health.

DH (2010a) *Equity and excellence: Liberating the NHS*, London: Department of Health.

DH (2010b) *Recognised, Valued, Supported: Next steps for the Carers Strategy*, London: Department of Health.

DH (2011) 'Personalised Care Planning Information Sheet 1', www.dh.gov.uk/longtermconditions.

Derrida, J. (2001) *Jacques Derrida: Deconstruction Engaged: The Sydney Seminars*, edited by P. Patton and T. Smith, Sydney: Power Publica.

Drew, N., Funk, M., Tang, S. et al (2011) 'Human rights violations of people with mental and psychosocial disabilities: an unresolved global crisis', *The Lancet,* vol 378, pp 1664–75, DOI 10.1016/S0140-6736(11)61458-X.

Du Preez, C.J. (2011) 'Living and care arrangements of non-urban households in KwaZulu-Natal, South Africa, in the context of HIV and AIDS', PhD thesis, Wageningen University, the Netherlands.

Du Preez, C.J. and Niehof, A. (2008) 'Caring for people living with AIDS. A labour of love', *Medische Antropologie*, vol 20, no 1, pp 87–105.

Du Preez, C.J. and Niehof, A. (2010) 'Impacts of AIDS-related morbidity and mortality on non-urban households in KwaZulu-Natal, South Africa', in A. Niehof, G. Rugalema and S. Gillespie (eds) *AIDS and Rural Livelihoods: Dynamics and Diversity in sub-Saharan Africa*, London: Earthscan, pp 43–61.

Dubois, C.A., McKee, M. and Nolte, E. (eds) (2006) *Human Resources for Health in Europe*, Berkshire: Open University Press.

Durie, M. (2001) *Mauri Ora: The Dynamics of Māori Health,* Auckland: Oxford University Press.

Ehn, B. and Löfgren, O. (2009) 'Routines – made and unmade', in E. Shove, F. Trentmann and R. Wilk (eds) *Time, Consumption and Everyday Life: Practice, Materiality and Culture*, Oxford and New York: Berg, pp 99–114.

Elder, G.S. (2003) *Hostels, Sexuality, and the Apartheid Legacy: Malevolent Geographies*, Ohio: Ohio University Press.

Elias, J. (2010) 'Gendered political economy and the politics of migrant worker rights: the view from South-East Asia', *Australian Journal of International Affairs*, vol 64, pp 70–85.

Elks, M.A. (2005) 'Visual indictment: A contextual analysis of *The Kallikak Family* photographs', *Mental Retardation*, vol 43, no 4, pp 268–80.

Emerson, E., Mallam, S., Davies, I. and Spencer, K. (2005) *Adults with Learning Disabilities in England 2003/2004*, London: Office for National Statistics and NHS Health and Social Care Information Centre.

Emond, R. (2003) 'Putting the Care into Residential Care: The Role of Young People', *Journal of Social Work*, vol 3, no 3, pp 321–37.

Emond, R. (2012) 'Longing to belong: children in residential care and their experiences of peer relationships at school and in the children's home', *Child and Family Social Work*, DOI 10.111/j.1365-2206.2012.00893.x.

England, K. and Henry, C. (2013) 'Care work, migration and citizenship: international nurses in the UK', *Social & Cultural Geography*, vol 14, pp 558–74.

Engster, D. (2005) 'Rethinking care theory: the practice of caring and the obligation to care', *Hypatia*, vol 20, no 3, pp 50–74.

Engster, D. (2007) *The Heart of Justice: Care ethics and political theory*, Oxford: Oxford University Press.

Escobar, A. (1995 [2012]) *Encountering Development: The Making and Unmaking of the Third World*, Princeton, NJ: Princeton University Press.

Escobar, A. (2001) 'Culture sits in places: Reflections on globalism and subaltern strategies of localization', *Political Geography*, vol 20, pp 139–74.

Esping-Andersen, G. (1990) *The Three Worlds of Welfare Capitalism*, Princeton NJ: Princeton University Press.

Esquith, S. (2010) *The Political Responsibilities of Everyday Bystanders*, University Park, PA: University of Pennsylvania Press.

Evans, R. (2011) '"We are managing our own lives …": Life transitions and care in sibling-headed households affected by AIDS in Tanzania and Uganda', *Area*, vol 43, no 4, pp 384–96.

Evans, R. (2012) 'Safeguarding inherited assets and enhancing the resilience of young people living in child- and youth-headed households in Tanzania and Uganda', *African Journal of AIDS Research*, vol 11, no 3, pp 177–89.

Evans, R. (2013) 'Young people's caring relations and transitions within families affected by HIV', in J. Ribbens McCarthy, C. Hooper and V. Gillies (eds) *Family Troubles? Exploring changes and challenges in the family lives of children and young people*, Bristol: Policy Press, 233–43.

Evans, R. and Atim, A. (2011) 'Care, Disability and HIV in Africa: diverging or interconnected concepts and practices?', *Third World Quarterly*, vol 32, no 8, pp 1437–54.

Evans, R. and Becker, S. (2009) *Children Caring for Parents with HIV and AIDS: Global Issues and Policy Responses*, Bristol: The Policy Press.

Evans, R. and Thomas, F. (2009) 'Emotional interactions and an ethic of care: caring relations in families affected by HIV and AIDS', *Emotions, Space and Society*, vol 2, pp 111–19.

Ferlander, S. (2007) 'The importance of different forms of social capital for health', *Acta Sociologica*, vol 50, no 2, pp 115–28.

Finch, J. and Mason, J. (1993) *Negotiating Family Responsibilities*, London: Routledge.

Fine, M. and Glendinning, C. (2005) 'Dependence, independence or inter-dependence? Revising the concepts of "care" and "dependency"', *Ageing and Society*, vol 25, pp 601–21.

Fineman, M.A. (2004) *The Autonomy Myth: A theory of dependency*, New York: The New Press.

Fish, J. (2006) *Heterosexism in Health and Social Care*, Basingstoke: Palgrave Macmillan.

Fisher, J.A. (2003) 'Curtailing the use of restraint in psychiatric settings', *Journal of Humanistic Psychology*, vol 43, pp 69–95.

Fisher, B. and Tronto, J.C. (1990) 'Toward a Feminist Theory of Caring', in E.K. Abel and M. Nelson (eds) *Circles of Care*, Albany, NY: State University of New York Press.

Folgheraiter, F. (2007) *Relational Social Work. Towards Networking and Societal Practices*, London: Jessica Kingsley.

Forrester, D. (2008) 'Is the care system failing children?', *The Political Quarterly*, vol 79, pp 206–11.

Foucault, M. (1964) *Madness and Civilisation: A history of insanity in the age of reason*, New York: Routledge.

Foucault, M. (1982) 'Afterword: The subject and power', in H.L. Dreyfuss and P. Rabinow (eds) *Michel Foucualt: Beyond structuralism and hermeneutics*, Chicago: University of Chicago Press.

Francis, R. (2013) *Report of the Mid Staffordshire NHS Foundation Trust Public Inquiry* Executive Summary, London: The Stationery Office, www.midstaffspublicinquiry.com/sites/default/files/report/Executive%20summary.pdf.

Frankenberg, R. (1993) *The Social Construction of Whiteness: White Women, Race Matters*, London: Routledge.

Fraser, N. (1997) *Justice Interruptus: Critical Reflections on the 'Postsocialist' Condition*, London and New York: Routledge.

Fraser, N. (2009) *Scales of Justice*, New York: Columbia University Press.

Freeman, J. (2011) 'From coercion to connection: Shifting an organisational culture', *Relational Child and Youth Care Practice*, vol 24, pp 128–32.

Fudge Schormans, A. (2011) 'The right or responsibility of inspection: Photography, social work, and people with intellectual disabilities', PhD thesis, University of Toronto.

Fudge Schormans, A. (2014) '"Weightless?": disrupting relations of power in/through photographic imagery of persons with intellectual disabilities', *Disability & Society*, vol 29, no 5, pp 699–713.

Fudge Schormans, A. (2015) 'Corroding the comforts of social work knowing: Persons with intellectual disabilities claim the right of inspection over public photographic images', in C. Sinding and H. Barnes (eds) *Social Work Beyond Borders/Social Work Artfully*, Waterloo, Ontario: Wilfrid Laurier University Press, pp 173–88.

Fudge Schormans, A. and Chambon, A. (2012) 'The re-working of spatial attribution: People with intellectual disabilities and the micropolitics of dissensus', *Review of Education, Pedagogy, & Cultural Studies*, vol 34, nos 3–4, pp 123–35.

Garfat, T. (2008) 'The inter-personal in-between: An exploration of relational child care practice', in G.Bellefeuille and F. Ricks (eds) *Standing on the precipice: Inquiry into the creative potential of child and youth care practice*, Alberta: MacEwan, pp 7–34.

Garland-Thomson, R. (2001) 'Seeing the disabled: Visual rhetorics of disability in popular photography', in eds P.K. Longmore and L. Umansky (eds) *The New Disability History: American Perspectives*, New York: New York University Press, pp 335–74.

Gasper, D. and Truong, T.D. (2010) 'Development ethics through the lens of caring, gender, and human security', in S. Esquith and F. Gifford (eds) *Capabilities, Power and Institutions: Toward a More Critical Development Ethics*, University Park, Pennsylvania: Pennsylvania State University Press, pp 58–95.

Gastmans, C. and Milisen, K. (2006) 'Use of physical restraint in nursing homes: clinical-ethical considerations', *Journal of Medical Ethics*, vol 32, pp 148–52.

Gervais, C. (2014) 'Suicide à l'hôpital: les anesthésistes réagissent', *La Nouvelle République*, 19 March, www.lanouvellerepublique.fr/Indre/Actualite/Faits-divers-justice/n/Contenus/Articles/2014/03/19/Suicide-a-l-hopital-les-anesthesistes-reagissent-1835675 (accessed 15 July 2014).

Giddens, A. (1996) *The Constitution of Society: Outline of the Theory of Structuration*, Berkeley, CA: University of California Press.

Gifford, H. and Boulton, A. (forthcoming) 'Is sharing tobacco within the home really good manaakitanga?', in M. Kepa, M. Brewin and L. Manu'atu (eds) *Home: Here to Stay*, Wellington: Huia Publications.

Gilligan, C. (1982) *In a Different Voice: Women's conceptions of voice and morality,* Cambridge, MA: Harvard University Press.

Gilligan, C. (1993) *In a Different Voice: Psychological Theory and Women's Development,*Cambridge, MA: Harvard University Press.

Gilligan, C. and Pollak, S. (1988) 'The vulnerable and invulnerable physicians', in C. Gilligan, J.V. Ward and J. McLean Taylor (eds) *Mapping the Moral Domain*, Cambridge, MA: Harvard University Press, pp 245–63.

Gilmour, J. and Brannelly, T. (2010) 'Representations of people with dementia – subaltern, person, citizen', *Nursing Inquiry*, vol 17, no 3, pp 240–7.

GMC (General Medical Council) (2013) *The State of Medical Education and Practice in the UK*, London: GMC.

Goffman, E. (1961) *Asylums: Essays on the social situation of mental patients and other inmates*, Harmondsworth: Penguin.

Gott, R. (2011) *Britain's Empire: Resistance, Repression and Revolt*, London: Verso.

Goulet, D. (1971 [1985]) *The Cruel Choice*, Lanham, MD: University Press of America.

Green, R.M., Mann, B. and Story, A.E. (2006) 'Care, domination, and representation', *Journal of Mass Media Ethics,* vol 21 no 2–3, pp 177–95.

Grootegoed, E. (2013) 'Between "choice" and "active citizenship": competing agendas for home care in the Netherlands', *Ethics and Social Welfare*, vol 7, no 2, pp 198–213.

Hage, G. (2000) *White Nation: Fantasies of White supremacy in a multicultural society*, New York: Routledge.

Hage, G. (2003) *Against Paranoid Nationalism,* Annandale, New South Wales: Pluto Press Australia.

Hall, S. and O'Shea, A. (2013) 'Common-sense neoliberalism', *Soundings*, vol 55, Winter, pp 8–24.

Hall, S. (1996) 'Introduction: who needs identity?', in S. Hall and P. du Gay (eds) *Questions of Cultural Identity*, London: Sage.

Halwani, R. (2003) 'Care ethics and virtue ethics', *Hypatia*, vol 18, no 3, pp 161–92.

Hankivsky, O. (2004) *Social Policy and the Ethic of Care*, Vancouver: University of British Columbia Press.

Hankivsky, O. (2006) 'Imagining ethical globalization: the contributions of a care ethic', *Journal of Global Ethics*, vol 2, no 1, pp 91–110.

Hankivsky, O. (2014) 'Rethinking care ethics: on the promise and potential of an intersectional analysis', *American Political Science Review,* vol 108, no 2, pp 252–64.

Hardy, K. (2001) 'African American experience and the healing of relationships', in D. Denborough (ed) *Family Therapy: Exploring the Field's Past, Present and Possible Futures*, Adelaide: Dulwich Centre Publications.

Harrison, G. (2005) 'Economic faith, social project, and a misreading of African society: The travails of neoliberalism in Africa', *Third World Quarterly*, vol 26, no 8, pp 1303–20.

Hart, D. and Howell, S. (2004) *Report on the Use of Physical Intervention across Children's Services*, London: National Children's Bureau.

Hart, S. (2009) 'The "problem" with youth: young people, citizenship and the community', *Citizenship Studies*, vol 13, pp 6, 641–57.

Hasmanová Marhánková, J. (2011) 'Leisure in old age: disciplinary practices surrounding the discourse of active ageing', *International Journal of Ageing and Later Life*, vol 6, no 1, pp 5–32.

HCPC (2013) 'Consultation on service user involvement in education and training programmes approved by the Health and Care Professions Council (HCPC)', www.hcpc-uk.org/assets/documents/10004110C onsultationonserviceuserinvolvementineducationandtrainingprogram mes-consultationresponsesanddecisions.pdf (accessed 9 August 2014).

Hekman, S.J. (1999) *The Future of Differences: Truth and method in feminist theory*, Cambridge: Polity Press.

Held, V. (2006) *The Ethics of Care: Personal, Political and Global*, Oxford: Oxford University Press.

Held, V. (2008) *How Terrorism is Wrong: Morality and Political Violence*, New York: Oxford University Press.

Held, V. (2010) 'Can the ethics of care handle violence?', *Ethics and Social Welfare*, vol 4, no 2, pp 115–29.

Helin, C. (2006) *Dances with Dependency: Indigenous success through self-reliance*, Vancouver: Orca Spirit Publishing and Communications Inc.

Helman, C.G. (2007) *Culture, Health and Illness*, 5th edn, New York: Oxford University Press.

Heron, G. (2006) 'Evidence-based policies for residential childcare staff: Who benefits from a minimalist approach to education and training?', *Evidence and Policy*, vol 2, pp 47–62.

Hevey, D. (1997) 'The enfreakment of photography', in L.J. Davis (ed) *The Disability Studies Reader*, New York: Routledge, pp 332–47.

Heymann, J. (2006) *Forgotten Families: Ending the Growing Crisis Confronting Children and Working Parents in the Global Economy*, New York: Oxford.

Heymann, J. and McNeill, K. (2012) 'Families at work: what we know about conditions globally', *United Nations Expert Group Meeting*, New York: United Nations Department of Economic and Social Affairs, Division for Social Policy and Development.

Higgs, P., Leontowitsch, M., Stevenson, F. and Jones, I.R. (2009) 'Not just old and sick – the "will to health", in later life', *Ageing and Society*, vol 10, no 5, pp 687–707.

Hines, S. (2007) 'Transgender care: practices of care in transgender communities', *Critical Social Policy*, vol 27, no 4, pp 462–86.

Hirschmann, N.J. (2002) *The Subject of Liberty: Toward a Feminist Theory of Freedom*, Princeton, NJ, Princeton University Press.

HMG (HM Government) (2010) *Healthy Lives, Healthy People: Our strategy for public health in England*, London: The Stationery Office.

Hochschild, A.R. (2000) 'Global care chains and emotional surplus value', in W. Hutton, A. Giddens (eds) *On The Edge: Living with Global Capitalism*, London: Jonathan Cape.

Hochschild, A.R. (2005) *The Chauffeur's Dilemma*, www.prospect.org/web/page.ww?section=root&name=ViewPrint&articleId=9877.

Holland, S. (2010) 'Looked after children and the ethic of care', *British Journal of Social Work*, vol 40, no 6, pp 1664–80.

Hollway, W. (2006) *The Capacity to Care: Gender and Ethical Subjectivity*, Hove: Routledge.

Holman, A., Rank, E., Ward, N.J. and West, R. (2009) *Sharing the Caring: Finding out about the support for carers for people with learning disabilities*, London: PRTC and Crossroads.

Holstein, M.B. and Minkler, M. (2003) 'Self, society and the "new gerontology"', *The Gerontologist*, vol 43, no 6, pp 787–96

Honderich, T. (1995) *The Oxford Companion to Philosophy*, New York: Oxford University Press.

Honneth, A. (1995) *The Struggle for Recognition: The moral grammar of social conflicts*, Cambridge: Polity Press.

Honneth, A. (2001) 'Invisibility. On the epistemology of "recognition"', *The Aristotelian Society*, supplementary vol, LXXV, pp 111–26.

Honneth, A. (2004) 'Recognition and justice: Outline of a plural theory of justice', *Acta Sociologica*, vol 47, no 4, pp 351–64.

Honneth, A. (2007) *Disrespect: The Normative Foundation of Critical Theory*, Cambridge: Polity Press.

hooks, b. (1991) *Yearning: Race, Gender and Cultural Politics*, London: Turnaround.

Hughes, B., McKie, L., Hopkins, D. and Watson, N. (2005) 'Love's labours lost? Feminism, the disabled people's movement and an ethic of care', *Sociology*, vol 39, pp 259–75.

Hutchings, A. and Buijs, G. (2005) 'Water and AIDS: problems associated with home-based care of AIDS patients in a rural area of Northern KwaZulu-Natal, South Africa', in A. Coles and T. Walace (eds) Gender, *Water and Development*, Oxford: Berg Publishers, pp 173–88.

ICDP (International Child Development Programme) (2008) *ICDP: Report 2008*, www.ucn.dk/Admin/Public/Download.aspx?file=Files%2FFiler%2FMicrosite%2FICDP%2FAnnual_report_2008_-_ICDP.pdf.

ICDP (2009) *Stories and Comments from Some of the ICDP Projects in the World*, www.icdp.info/var/uploaded/2013/04/2013-04-06_10-30-12_storiesfromprojects.pdf.

ICDP (2010) *ICDP: International Child Development Programme: Empathy in Action: ICDP in the World 2010*, www.icdp.info/var/uploaded/2013/04/2013-04-10_05-13-50_annualreport2010.pdf.

IDS (Institute for Development Studies) (2004) 'Immersions for policy and personal change', *IDS Policy Briefing* no 22, www.ids.ac.uk/files/PB22.pdf.

International Labour Organisation (2013) *The Founding Congress of the IDWF*, Available at:http://www.ilo.org/wcmsp5/groups/public/@ed_protect/@protrav/@migrant/documents/newsitem/wcms_232879.pdf

Isin, E.F. (2008) 'Theorising acts of citizenship', in E.F. Isin and G.M. Nielsen (eds) *Acts of Citizenship*, London: Zed Books.

Jackson, M. (2010) 'Constitutional transformation: an interview with Moana Jackson', in M. Mulholland and V. Tawhai (eds) *Weeping Waters: The Treaty of Waitangi and Constitutional Change*, Wellington: Huia Publishers.

Jawad, R. (2012) *Religion and Faith-based Welfare: From wellbeing to ways of being*, Bristol: Policy Press.

Kamp, A. and Hvid, H. (eds) (2012) *Elderly Care in Transition*, Copenhagen: Copenhagen Business School Press.

Katz, S. (2000) 'Busy bodies: activity, aging, and the management of everyday life', *Journal of Aging Studies*, vol 14, no 2, pp 135–52.

Kawharu, M. (2000) 'Kaitiakitanga: A Māori anthropological perspective of the Māori socio-environmental ethic of resource management', *The Journal of the Polynesian Society*, vol 109, no 4, pp 349–70.

Kendall, E. and Rogers, A. (2007) 'Extinguishing the social? state sponsored self-care policy and the Chronic Disease Self-Management Programme', *Disability and Society*, vol 22, no 2, pp 129–43.

Kittay, E.F. (1999) *Love's Labor. Essays on Women, Equality and Dependency*, London and New York: Routledge.

Kittay, E.F. (2001a) 'A feminist public ethic of care meets the new communitarian family policy', *Ethics*, vol 111, no 3, pp 523–47.

Kittay, E. (2001b) 'When caring is just and justice is caring: Justice and mental retardation', *Public Culture,* vol 13, pp 557–79.

Kittay, E. (2002a) 'Love's labor revisited', *Hypatia*, vol 17, no 3, pp 237–50.

Kittay, E.F (2002b) 'When caring is just and justice is caring: justice and mental retardation', in E.F. Kittay and E. Feder (eds) *The Subject of Care: Feminist Perspectives on Dependency,* Lanham, MD: Rowman and Littlefield, pp 257–76.

Kittay, E.F. (2010) 'The personal is philosophical is political: a philosopher and mother of a cognitively disabled person sends notes from the battlefield', in E.F. Kittay and L. Carlson (eds) *Cognitive Disability and its Challenge to Moral Philosophy*, Chichester: Wiley-Blackwell, pp 393–413.

Kittay, E.F. and Carlson, L. (eds) (2010) *Cognitive Disability and its Challenge to Moral Philosophy*, Chichester: Wiley-Blackwell.

Koggel, C.M. (2006) 'Global inequalities and relational ethics', *Annual Meeting of the American Political Science Association*, Philadelphia, PA: American Political Science Association.

Koggel, C.M. (2008) 'Ecological thinking and epistemic location: the local and the global', *Hypatia*, vol 23, no 1, pp 177–86.

Koggel, C.M. (2009) 'Agency and empowerment: embodied realities in a globalized world', in S. Campbell and L. Meynell (eds) *Embodiment and Agency*, State College PA: Penn State Press, pp 250–69.

Koggel, C. and Orme, J. (2010) 'Care ethics: new theories and applications', *Ethics and Social Welfare*, vol 4, no 2, pp 109–14.

Kröger, T. (2009) 'Care research and disability studies: Nothing in common?', *Critical Social Policy*, vol 29, no 3, pp 398–420.

Laliberte Rudman, D. (2006) 'Shaping the active, autonomous and responsible modern retiree: an analysis of discursive technologies and their links with neo-liberal political rationality', *Ageing & Society*, vol 26, pp 181–201.

Lancioni, G.E., Cuvo, A.J. and O'Reilly, M.F. (2002) 'Snoezelen: an overview of research with people with developmental disabilities and dementia', *Disability and Rehabilitation*, vol 24, pp 175–84.

Lanoix, M. (2007) 'The citizen in question', *Hypatia*, vol 22, no 4, pp 113–29.

Laslett, P. (1989) *A Fresh Map of Life: The Emergence of the Third Age*, London: Weidenfeld and Nicolson.

Layder, D. (2004) *Social and Personal Identity: Understanding yourself*, London: Sage.

Lemon, R. (no date) 'The impact of new media on Māori culture and belief systems', unpublished paper, Te Ara Poutama, Faculty of Māori Development, Auckland University of Technology, Auckland.

Le Roux, T. (1995) *"We have Families Too": Live-in domestics talk about their lives*, Pretoria: Human Sciences Research Council.

Levin, E. (2004) *Involving Service Users and Carers in Social Work Education*, London: Social Care Institute for Excellence.

Levitas, R. (2012) 'The just's umbrella: Austerity and the Big Society in Coalition policy and beyond', *Critical Social Policy*, vol 32, pp 320–42.

Lewis, G. (1998) 'Citizenship', in G. Hughes (ed) *Imagining welfare futures*, London: Routledge/Open University Press, pp 103–50.

Li, C. (2008) 'Does Confucian ethics integrate care ethics and justice ethics? the case of Mencius', *Asian Philosophy*, vol 18, no 1, pp 69–82.

Lister, R. (2003) *Citizenship: Feminist Perspectives*, Basingstoke: Macmillan.

Lister, R., Williams, F., Antonnen, A., Bussemaker, M., Gerhard, U., Johansson, S., Heinen, J., Leira, A., Siim, B., Tobio, C. and Gavanas, A. (2007) *Gendered citizenship in Western Europe: new challenges for citizenship research in a cross-national context*, Bristol: Policy Press.

Liveng, A. and Andersen, H.L. (2011) *Fra Dagtilbud til Aktivitetstilbud*, http://rucforsk.ruc.dk/admin/editor/dk/atira/pure/api/shared/model/base_dk/cust_dk_ruc/publication/editor/bookanthologyeditor.xhtml.

Lloyd, L. (2004) 'Mortality and morality: ageing and the ethic of care', *Ageing and Society*, vol 24, pp 235–56.

Lloyd, L. (2010) 'The individual in Social Care: The Ethics of Care and the "Personalisation Agenda", in Services for Older People in England', *Ethics and Social Welfare*, vol 4, no 2, pp 188–200.

Lloyd, L. (2012) *Health and Care in Ageing Societies: A new international approach*, Bristol: Policy Press.

Lloyd, L., Calnan, M., Cameron, A. et al (2012) 'Identity in the fourth age: perseverance, adaptation and maintaining dignity', *Ageing and Society*, vol 34, no 1, pp 1–19.

Lopez, D. (2010) 'The securitization of care spaces: lessons from telecare', in M. Schillmeyer and M. Domènech (eds) *New Technologies and Emerging Spaces of Care*, New York: Ashgate, pp 39–56.

Lutz, H. (2011) *The New Maids: Transnational Women and the Care Economy*, New York: Zed Books.

Lynch, K., Baker, J. et al (eds) (2009) *Affective Equality: Love, Care and Injustice*, Basingstoke: Palgrave Macmillan.

McCarthy, J.R. (2013) 'Caring after death. Issues of embodiment and relationality', in C. Rogers and S. Weller (eds) *Critical Approaches to Care. Understanding caring relations, identities and cultures*, London: Routledge.

McDowell, L. (2004) 'Work, workfare, work/life balance and an ethic of care', *Progress in human Geography*, vol 28, no 2, pp 145–63.

McEwan, C. and Goodman, M.K. (2010) 'Place geography and the ethics of care: introductory remarks on the geographies of ethics, responsibility and care', *Ethics, Policy and Environment*, vol 13, no 2, pp 103–12.

McIlwaine, C. (2007) 'From local to global to transnational civil society: reframing development perspectives on the non-state sector', *Geography Compass*, vol 1, no 6, pp 1252–81.

McIntosh, P. (2010) 'White privilege and male privilege: a personal account of coming to see correspondences through work in women's studies', in M.S. Kimmel and A.L. Ferber (eds) *Privilege. A Reader*, 2nd edn, Boulder, CO: Westview Press.

Mackay, F. (2001) *Love and Politics: Women politicians and the ethics of care*, London and New York: Continuum.

MacKenzie, C. and Stoljar, N. (eds) (2000) *Relational Autonomy: Feminist Perspectives on Autonomy, Agency and the Social Self*, Oxford: Oxford University Press.

McKie, L., Gregory, S. and Bowlby, S. (2002) 'Shadow times: the temporal and spatial frameworks and experiences of caring and working', *Sociology*, vol 36, no 4, pp 897–924.

McNatty, W. and Roa, T. (2002) 'Whanaungatanga: An Illustration of the Importance of Cultural Context', *He Puna Korero: Journal of Māori and Pacific Development*, vol 3, no 1, pp 88–96.

McPheat, G., Milligan, I. and Hunter, L. (2007) 'What's the use of residential childcare? Findings of two studies detailing current trends in the use of residential childcare in Scotland', *Journal of Children's Services*, vol 2, pp 15–25.

Madoerin, K. (2008) *Mobilising Children and Youth into their Own Child- and Youth-led Organisations*, Johannesburg, South Africa: Regional Psychosocial Support Initiative.

Mahon, R. and Robinson, F. (2011) *Feminist Ethics and Social Policy: Towards a new global political economy of care*, Vancouver: University of British Columbia Press.

Makina, A. (2009) 'Caring for people with HIV: State policies and their dependence on women's unpaid work', *Gender and Development*, vol 17, no 2, pp 309–19.

Manea, T. (2011) 'Romanian medical migration: an issue of trust?', *Romanian Journal of Bioethics*, vol 9, no 3, pp 61–2.

Marcia, J. (1987) 'Empathy and psychotherapy', in N. Eisenberg and J. Strayer (eds) *Empathy and its development*, pp 81–102, New York: Cambridge University Press.

Marsden, M. and Henare, T.A. (1992) *Kaitiakitanga: A Definitive Introduction to the Holistic Worldview of the Māori*, Wellington: Ministry for the Environment.

Marshall, T.H. (1950) *Citizenship and Social Class*, Cambridge: Cambridge University Press.

Massey, D. (2013) 'Vocabularies of the economy', in S. Hall, D. Massey and M. Ruskin (eds) *After Neoliberalism? The Kilburn Manifesto*, www.lwbooks.co.uk.

Mead, H.M. (2003) *Tikanga Maori, Living by Maori Values*, Wellington: Huia Press.

Meagher, G. and Parton, N. (2004) 'Modernising social work and the ethics of care', *Social Work and Society*, vol 2, pp 10–27.

Miers, M. (2002) 'Developing an understanding of gender sensitive care: exploring concepts and knowledge', *Journal of Advanced Nursing*, vol 40, no 1, pp 69–77.

Miller, M.N. and Mcgowen, K.R. (2000) 'The painful truth: physicians are not invincible', *Southern Medical Journal*, vol 93, no 10, pp 966–72.

Minhinnick, N. (1989) *Establishing Kaitiaki: A paper*, Auckland: Nganeko Kaihau Minhinnick.

Ministry of Health (2013) *Office of the Director of Mental Health Annual Report for 2012*, Wellington: Ministry of Health.

Misra, J., Woodring, J. and Merz, S. (2006) 'The globalization of care work: Neoliberal economic restructuring and migration policy', *Globalizations*, vol 3, pp 317–32.

Mol, A. (2008) *The Logic of Care: Health and the Problem of Patient Choice*, London and New York: Routledge.

Mol, A., Moser, I. and Pols, J. (2010) *Care in Practice. On Tinkering in Clinics, Homes and Farms*, Bielefeld: Transcript Verlag.

Molyneux, M. (2002) 'Gender and the silences of social capital: Lessons from Latin America', *Development and Change*, vol 33, pp 167–88.

Montgomery, C.M., Hosegood, V., Busza, J. and Timæs, I.M. (2006) 'Men's involvement in the South African family: Engendering change in the AIDS era', *Social Science & Medicine*, vol 62, pp 2411–19.

Moran, N., Glendinning, C., Wilberforce, M., Stevens, M., Netten, A., Jones, K., Manthorpe, J., Knapp, M., Fernandez, J-L., Challis, D. and Jacobs, S. (2013) 'Older people's experiences of cash-for-care schemes: evidence from the English individual budget pilot projects', *Ageing & Society*, vol 33, no 5, pp 826–51.

Morgan, R. (2012) 'Children's views on restraint', www.crisisprevention. com/CPI/media/Media/Resources/KnowledgeBase/Childrens-views-on-restraint-2012.pdf.

Morrell, M. (2010) *Empathy and Democracy: Feeling, Thinking and Deliberation*, University Park, PA: University of Pennsylvania Press.

Morris, J. (1991) *Pride Against Prejudice: Transforming Attitudes to Disability*, Philadelphia: New Society Publishers.

Morris, J. (2001) 'Impairment and disability: constructing an ethics of care that promotes human rights', *Hypatia*, vol 16, no 4, pp 1–16.

Morris, J. (2004) 'Independent living and community care: a disempowering framework', *Disability and Society*, vol 19, no 5, pp 427–42.

Morris, J. (2011) *Rethinking Disability Policy*, York: Joseph Rowntree Foundation.

Mort, M. et al (2013) 'Ethical implications of home telecare for older people: a framework derived from a multi-sited participative study', *Health Expectations*, DOI 10.1111/hex.12109.

Moser, I. (2006) 'Disability and the promises of technology: Technology, subjectivity and embodiment within an order of the normal', *Information, Communication and Society*, vol 9, pp 373–95.

Moser, I. (2011) 'Dementia and the limits to life: Anthropological sensibilities, STS interferences, and possibilities for action in care', *Science, Technology & Human Values*, vol 36, no 5, pp 704–22.

Moss, P. and Petrie, P. (2002) *From Children's Services to Children's Spaces: Public policy, children and childhood*, London: Routledge Falmer.

Mtshali, S.M. (2002) 'Household livelihood security in rural KwaZulu-Natal, South Africa', PhD thesis, Wageningen University, The Netherlands.

Munro, E. (2011) *The Munro Review of Child Protection: Final Report*, London: Department for Education.

Nare, L. (2013) 'The ethics of transnational market familism: inequalities and hierarchies in the Italian elderly care', *Ethics and Social Welfare*, vol 7, no 2, pp 184–97.

National Task Force on Violence Against Social Care Staff (2000) *Report and National Action Plan*, London: National Task Force on Violence Against Social Care Staff.

Needham, C. (2014) 'Personalization: From day centres to community hubs?', *Critical Social Policy*, vol 34, no 1, pp 90–108.

Needham, C. and Carr, S. (2009) *SCIE Research briefing 31: Co-production: an emerging evidence base for adult social care transformation*, London: Social Care Institute for Excellence.

NHS (2004) *Code of Practice for the International Recruitment of Healthcare Professionals*, www.dh.gov.uk/en/Publicationsandstatistics/ Publications/PublicationsPolicyAndGuidance/DH_4097730.

NHS (2013) www.imsrecruitment.com/nhs_doctor_jobs.html (accessed 10 December 2013).

Niehof, A. (2004) 'A micro-ecological approach to home care for AIDS patients', *Medische Antropologie*, vol 16, no 2, pp 245–66.

Niehof, A. (2012) 'HIV/AIDS in sub-Saharan Africa: impacts and social change', *Afriche e Orienti, Special issue on AIDS 2012* [Bologna], pp 36–46.

Noddings, N. (1984) *Caring: A Feminine Approach to Ethics and Moral Education*, Berkeley, CA: University of California Press.

Noddings, N. (1996a) 'The Cared-For', in S. Gordon, P. Benner and N. Noddings (eds) *Caregiving: Readings in Knowledge, Practice, Ethics and Politics*, Philadelphia: University of Pennsylvania Press, pp 21–39.

Noddings, N. (1996b) 'The caring professional', in S. Gordon, P. Benner and N. Noddings (eds) *Caregiving: Readings in Knowledge, Practice, Ethics and Politics*, Philadelphia: University of Pennsylvania Press, pp 160–72.

Nombo, C.I. (2007) *When AIDS meets Poverty: Implications for Social Capital in a Village in Tanzania*, AWLAE Series 5, Wageningen: Wageningen Academic Publishers.

Nombo, C.I. (2010) 'Sweet cane, bitter realities: The complex realities of AIDS in Mkamba, Kilombero District, Tanzania', in A. Niehof, G. Rugalema and S. Gillespie (eds) *AIDS and Rural Livelihoods: Dynamics and Diversity in sub-Saharan Africa*, London: Earthscan, pp 61–76.

Nombo, C.I. and Niehof, A. (2008) 'Resilience of HIV/AIDS-affected households in a village in Tanzania: Does social capital help?', *Medische Antropologie*, vol 20, no 2, pp 241–59.

Nussbaum, M. (1995) 'Human capabilities, female human beings', in M. Nussbaum and J. Glover (eds) *Women, Culture and Development. A study of human capabilities*, Oxford: Clarendon Press.

Nussbaum, M. (2001) *Women and Human Development: The Capabilities Approach*, Cambridge: Cambridge University Press.

Nussbaum, M.C. (2003) 'Capabilities as fundamental entitlements: Sen and social justice', *Feminist Economics*, vol 9, nos 2–3, pp 33–59.

Nussbaum, M. (2011) *Creating Capabilities: The Human Development Approach*, Cambridge, MA: Belknap Press.

Oakley Browne, M.A., Wells, J.E. and Scott, K.M. (eds) (2006) *Te Rau Hinengaro The New Zealand Mental Health Survey*, Wellington: Ministry of Health.

O'Carroll, A.D. (2013) 'Virtual whanaungatanga: Māori utilizing social networking sites to attain and maintain relationships', *AlterNative: An International Journal of Indigenous Peoples*, vol 9, no 3, pp 230–45.

Ogden, J., Esim, S. and Grown, C. (2006) 'Expanding the care continuum for HIV/AIDS: bringing carers into focus', *Health Policy and Planning*, vol 21, no 5, pp 333–42.

O'Hara, D.R. (2008) 'Disability and embodiment: Towards an ethics of welcoming', MA in Philosophy thesis, Stony Brook University.

Olthuis, G., Kohlen, H. and Heier, J. (eds) (2014) *Moral Boundaries Redrawn: The significance of Joan Tronto's argument for political theory, professional ethics and care as a practice*, Leuven: Peeters.

Omolade, B. (1994) *The Rising Song of African American Women*, New York and London: Routledge.

Owen, J.L. and Floyd, M. (2010) 'Negotiated coercion: thoughts about involuntary treatment in mental health', *Ethics and Social Welfare*, vol 4, no 3, pp 297–99.

Paradza, G.G. (2010) 'Single women's experiences of livelihood conditions, HIV and AIDS in the rural areas of Zimbabwe', in A. Niehof, G. Rugalema and S. Gillespie (eds) *AIDS and Rural Livelihoods: Dynamics and Diversity in sub-Saharan Africa*, London: Earthscan, pp 77–95.

Parreñas, R.S. (2001) *Servants of Globalization: Women, Migration, and Domestic Work,* Stanford, CA: Stanford University Press.

Parrenas, R. (2005) *Children of Global Migration: Transnational Families and Gendered Woes,* Stanford, CA: Stanford University Press.

Parton, N. (2003) 'Rethinking professional practice: The contributions of social constructionism and the feminist "ethics of care"', *British Journal of Social Work*, vol 33, pp 1–16.

Paterson, B., Leadbetter, D., Miller, G. and Crichton, J. (2008) 'Adopting a public health model to reduce violence and restraints in children's residential care facilities', in M.A. Nunno, D.M. Dayand, L.B. Bullard (eds) *For our own safety: Examining the safety of high-risk interventions for children and young people*, Arlington, VA: Child Welfare League of America, pp 127–41.

Paterson, S., Watson, D. and Whiteford, J. (2003) *Let's Face It! Care 2003: Young people tell us how it is*, Glasgow: Who Cares? Scotland.

Paulsen, J.E. (2011) 'A narrative ethics of care', *Health Care Analysis An International Journal of Health Care Philosophy and Policy*, DOI 10.1007/s10728-010-0162-8.

Peacock, D. and Weston, M. (2008) 'Men and care in the context of HIV and AIDS: Structure, political will and greater male involvement', New York: United Nations, Division for the Advancement of Women.

Pease, B. (2010) *Undoing Privilege: Unearned advantage in a divided world*, London: Zed Books.

Pease, B. (2011) 'Men in social work: Challenging or reproducing an unequal gender regime?', *Affilia: Journal of Women and Social Work*, vol 26, no 4, pp 406–18.

Pedwell, C. (2012) 'Affective (self-)transformations: Empathy, neoliberalism and international development', *Feminist Theory*, vol 13, no 2, pp 163–79.

Peters, H., Fiske, J., Hemingway, D., Vaillancourt, A., McLennan, C., Keith, B. and Burrill, A. (2010) 'Interweaving caring and economics in the context of place: experiences of Northern and rural women caregivers', *Ethics and Social Welfare*, vol 4, no 2, pp 172–87.

Pettersen, T. and Hem, M.H. (2011) 'Mature care and reciprocity: Two cases from acute psychiatry', *Nursing Ethics*, vol 18, no 2, pp 217–31.

Phillips, A. and Rakusen, J. (1978) (eds) *Our Bodies, Ourselves*, Harmondsworth: Penguin.

Plotnikova, E.V. (2012) 'Cross-border mobility of health professionals: Contesting patients' right to health', *Social Science and Medicine*, vol 74, pp 20–7.

Plumwood, V. (1993) *Feminism and the Mastery of Nature*, London and New York: Routledge.

Plumwood, V. (2002) *Environmental Culture: The Ecological Crisis of Reason*, London and New York: Routledge.

Pols, J. (2012) *Care at a Distance: On the closeness of technology*, Amsterdam: Amsterdam University Press.

Pols, J. (2014) 'Radical relationality. Epistemology in care, care ethics for research', in G. Olthuis et al (eds) *Moral Boundaries Redrawn. The Significance of Joan Tronto's argument for Political Theory, Professional Ethics and Care as Practice*, Leuven: Peeters Publishers, pp 175–94.

Pols J. and Moser, I. (2009) 'Cold technologies versus warm care? On affective and social relations with and through care technologies', *ALTER, European Journal of Disability, Research*, vol 3, no 2, pp 159–78.

Power, A. (2010) 'The geographies of interdependence in the lives of people with intellectual disabilities', in V. Chouinard, E. Hall and R. Wilton (eds) *Towards Enabling Geographies, 'Disabled Bodies and Minds in Society and Space*, Farnham: Ashgate, pp 107–22.

Price, E. (2010) 'Coming out to care: gay and lesbian carers' experiences of dementia services', *Health and Social Care in the Community*, vol 18, no 2, pp 160–68.

Pulcini, E. (2009) *Care of the World: Fear, Responsibility and Justice in the Global Age,* Dordrecht: Springer.

QAA (2000) *Benchmark statement for social work*, Gloucester: The Quality Assurance Agency for Higher Education.

Raghuram, P. (2009) 'Caring about "brain drain" migration in a postcolonial world', *Geoforum*, vol 40, pp 25–33.

Raghuram, P., Madge, C. and Naxolo, P. (2009) 'Rethinking responsibility and care in a postcolonial world', *Geoforum*, vol 40, pp 5–13.

Razavi, S. (2007) 'The political and social economy of care in a development context: Conceptual issues, research questions and policy options', *Gender and Development Programme Paper* no 3, Geneva: UNRISD.

Razavi, S. and Staab, S. (2012) *Global Variations in the Political and Social Economy of Care: Worlds Apart*, London: Routledge.

Ritchie, J.E. (1992) *Becoming bicultural*, Wellington: Huia Publishers and Daphne Brasell Associates Press.

Roa, T. and Tuaupiki, J.T. (2005) 'Tikanga Tainui; Tikanga Whare Wananga, Te Pua Wananga ki te Ao', University of Waikato, www.waikato.ac.nz/tekowhao/files/tikanga_tainui.pdf (accessed 24 July 2013).

Roberts, C. and Mort, M. (2009) 'Reshaping what counts as care: Older people, work and new technologies', *ALTER – European Journal of Disability Research*, vol 3, pp 138–58.

Robinson, F. (1999) *Globalizing Care: Ethics, Feminist theory and International Relations,* Colorado and Oxford: West View Press.

Robinson, F. (2006) 'Care, gender and global social justice: Rethinking "ethical globalization"', *Journal of Global Ethics*, vol 2, no 1, pp 5–25.

Robinson, F. (2011) *The Ethics of Care: A Feminist Approach to Human Security*, Philadelphia: Temple University Press.

Rose, D., Barnes, M., Crawford, M., Omeni, E., MacDonald, D. and Wilson, A. (2013) *How do managers and leaders in the National Health Service and social care respond to service user involvement in mental health services in both its traditional and emergent forms*, NIHR, www.journalslibrary.nihr.ac.uk/__data/assets/pdf_file/0015/117006/FullReport-hsdr02100.pdf.

Rowe, J.W. and Kahn, R.L. (1997) 'Successful Aging', *The Gerontologist*, vol 37, no 4, pp 433–40.

Royal, T.A.C. (2011) 'Preface', in T. McIntosh and M. Mulholland (eds) *Māori and Social Issues*, Wellington: Huia Publishers.

Ruch, G. (2011) 'Where have all the feelings gone? Developing reflective and relationship-based management in child-care social work', *British Journal of Social Work*, vol 42, no 7, pp 1315–32.

Rugkasa, J. and Burns, T. (2009) 'Community Treatment Orders', *Psychiatry*, vol 8, no 12, pp 493–5.

Saith, A. (2006) 'From universal values to Millennium Development Goals: Lost in translation', *Development and Change*, vol 37, no 6, pp 1167–99.

Sarkar, S. (2010) 'Community engagement in HIV prevention in Asia: going from "for the community" to "by the community" – must we wait for more evidence?', *Sexually Transmitted Infections*, vol 86, no 1, pp 2–3.

Sarti, R. (2005) 'Conclusion: Domestic service and European identity', in S. Pasleau and I. Schopp (eds) *Proceedings of the Servant Project*, Liege: Editions de l'Université de Liege, pp 195–285.

Sarti, R. (2006) 'Domestic Service: Past and Present in Southern and Northern Europe', *Gender & History*, vol 18, pp 222–45.

Sayer, A. (2011) *Why Things Matter to People: Social Science, Values and Ethical Life*, Cambridge: Cambridge University Press.

Schiele, J.H. (1996) 'Afrocentricity: An emerging paradigm in social work practice', *Social Work*, vol 41, no 3, pp 284–94.

Scottish Council Foundation (1999) *Children, Families and Learning: A new agenda for education*, Edinburgh: Children in Scotland and Scottish Council Foundation.

Scottish Institute of Residential Child Care (2010) 'Residential Child Care Qualifications Audit', www.celcis.org/media/resources/publications/RCC-Qualifications-Audit-2009.pdf.

Scuzzarello, S., Kinnvall, C. and Monroe, K.R. (eds) (2009) *On Behalf of Others. The Psychology of Care in a Global World,* Oxford: Oxford University Press.

Self-Care Forum (2013), www.selfcareforum.org/about-us/what-do-we-mean-by-self-care-and-why-is-good-for-people.

Sen, A.K. (1995) 'Gender inequality and theories of justice', in M. Nussbaum and J. Glover (eds) *Women, Culture and Development. A study of human capabilities*, Oxford: Clarendon Press, pp 259–73.

Sen, A.K. (1999) *Development as Freedom*, New York: Random House Ltd.

Sen, A.K. (2001) *Development as Freedom*, 2nd edn, Oxford and New York: Oxford University Press.

Sensoy, Ö. and DiAngelo, R. (2012) *Is Everyone Really Equal? An introduction to key concepts in social justice education*, New York: Teachers College Press.

Sevenhuijsen, S. (1998) *Citizenship and the Ethics of Care. Feminist Considerations on Justice, Morality and Politics*, London and New York: Routledge.

Sevenhuijsen, S. (2000) 'Caring in the third way: the relation between obligation, responsibility and care in Third Way discourse', *Critical Social Policy*, vol 20, no 1, pp 5–37.

Sevenhuijsen, S. (2003) 'The place of care. the relevance of the ethics of care for social policy', in S. Sevenhuijsen and A. Svab (eds) *Labyrinth of Care. The relevance of the ethics of care perspective for social policy*, Ljubljana: Mirovni Institut, pp 13–43.

Sevenhuijsen, S. (2004) 'TRACE: a method for normative policy analysis from the ethic of care', in S. Sevenhuijsen and A. Švab, *The Heart of the Matter: The Contribution of the Ethic of Care to Social Policy in some new EU Member States*, Ljubljana: Peace Institute, Institute for Contemporary Social and Political Studies.

Shachar, A. (2006) 'The race for talent: highly skilled migrants and competitive immigration regimes', *New York University Law Review*, vol 81, pp 148–233.

Shaikh, N. (2007) *The Present as History: Critical Perspectives on Global Power*, New York: Columbia University Press.

Shakespeare, T. (1993) 'Disabled people's self-organisation: a new social movement?', *Disability, Handicap and Society*, vol 8, no 3, pp 249–64.

Shakespeare, T. (2006) *Disability Rights and Wrongs*, London: Routledge.

Sharp, J. and Spiegel, A. (1990) 'Women and wages: gender and the control of income in farm and bantustan households', *Journal of Southern African Studies*, vol 16, no 3, pp 527–49.

Shawler, C. (2007) 'Empowerment of aging mothers and daughters in transition during a health crisis', *Qualitative Health Research*, vol 17, no 6, pp 838–49.

Sherr, L., Solheim Skar, A.-M., Clucas, C., von Tetzchner, S. and Hundeide, K. (2011) *Evaluation of the Parental Guidance Programme based on the International Child Development Programme. Report to the Ministry of Children, Equality, and Social Inclusion,* June 2011, www.regjeringen. no/globalassets/upload/bld/rapporter/2011/foreldreveiledning1.pdf (accessed 27 May 2013).

Sholock, A. (2012) 'Methodology of the privileged: White Anti-racist Feminism, Systematic Ignorance, and Epistemic Uncertainty', *Hypatia,* vol 27, no 4, pp 701–14.

Skelton, D.F. (2014) *Artisans of Peace Overcoming Poverty, volume 1: A People-Centred Movement,* published online by ATD Fourth World, full text available at: http://ebook.atd-fourthworld.org/ (accessed 7 October 2014).

Skelton, J.R., Kai, J. and Loudon, R.F. (2001) 'Cross-cultural communication in medicine: questions for educators', *Medical Education,* vol 35, no 3, pp 257–61.

Slote, M. (2007) *The Ethics of Care and Empathy,* Oxford: Oxford University Press.

Smith, L.T. (1999) *Decolonizing Methodologies: Research and indigenous peoples,* London: Zed Books.

Smith, M. (2009) *Rethinking Residential Child Care,* Bristol: Policy Press.

Smith, M., Fulcher, L.C. and Doran, P. (2013) *Residential Child Care In Practice: Making a difference,* Bristol: Policy Press.

Spiller, C., Erakovic, L., Henare, M. and Pio, E. (2011) 'Relational well-being and wealth: Māori businesses and an ethic of care', *Journal of Business Ethics,* vol 98, pp 153–69, DOI 10.1007/s10551-010-0540-z.

Steckley, L. (2009) 'Therapeutic containment and physical restraint in residential child care', *The Goodenoughcaring Journal,* 6, www.goodenoughcaring.com/Journal/Article110.htm.

Steckley, L. (2010) 'Containment and holding environments: Understanding and reducing physical restraint in residential child care', *Children and Youth Services Review,* vol 32, pp 120–8.

Steckley, L. (2012) 'Touch, physical restraint and therapeutic containment in residential child care', *British Journal of Social Work,* vol 42, pp 537–55.

Steckley, L. and Kendrick, A. (2008a) 'Hold on: Physical restraint in residential child care', in A. Kendrick (ed) *Residential child care: Prospects and challenges,* London: Jessica Kingsley, pp 152–65.

Steckley, L. and Kendrick, A. (2008b) 'Physical restraint in residential child care: The experiences of young people and residential workers', *Childhood,* vol 15, pp 552–69.

Steckley, L. and Kendrick, A. (2008c) 'Young people's experiences of physical restraint in residential care: subtlety and complexity in policy and practice', in M.A. Nunno, D.M. Dayand and L.B. Bullard (eds) *For Our Own Safety: Examining the Safety of High-risk Interventions for Children and Young People*, Washington, DC: Child Welfare League of America, pp 3–24.

Steckley, L. and Smith, M. (2011) 'Care ethics in residential child care: A different voice', *Ethics and Social Welfare*, vol 5, pp 181–95.

Stevens, I. (2008) 'Complexity theory: Developing new understandings of child protection in field settings and in residential child care', *British Journal of Social Work*, vol 38, pp 1320–36.

Strumpf, N.E. and Evans, L.K. (1991) 'The ethical problems of prolonged physical restraint', *Journal of Gerontological Nursing*, vol 17, pp 27–30.

Sullivan, S. (2006) *Revealing Whiteness: The unconscious habits of racial privilege*, Bloomington and Indianapolis: Indiana University Press.

Surrey and Borders NHS Partnership (2007) 'Intimate care policy', ref SABP/Service/improvements/0029, www.sabp.nhs.uk/aboutus/policies/G-I/SABP0029Intimate%20Care%20Policy%20for%20approvaljan%2007.pdf.

Swigonski, M.E. (1996) 'Challenging privilege through Africentric social work practice', *Social Work*, vol 41, no 2, pp 153–61.

Szasz, T.S. (1960) 'The myth of mental illness', *American Psychologist*, vol 15, no 2, pp 113–18.

Tache, S. and Schillinger, D. (2009) 'Health worker migration: time or the global justice approach', *The American Journal of Bioethics*, vol 9, no 3, pp 12–14.

Tanner, D. (2010) *Managing the Ageing Experience: Learning from older people*, Bristol: Policy Press.

Tanzania Country Report (2012) 'Country progress reporting. Part A: Tanzania Mainland. Dodoma: The United Republic of Tanzania' [UNAIDS Country Reports].

Taxis, J.C. (2002) 'Ethics and praxis: Alternative strategies to physical restraint and seclusion in a psychiatric setting', *Issues in Mental Health Nursing*, vol 23, pp 157–70.

Te Ara: The Encyclopedia of New Zealand, www.teara.govt.nz/en/taupori-maori-maori-population-change/page-1.

Teodorescu, C., Manea, T., Oprea, L. and Gavrilovici, C. (2013) 'International medical migration and the patient-physician relationship', *Romanian Journal of Bioethics*, vol 11, no 2, pp 77–87.

The Scottish Government (2013) *Children's Social Work Statistics: Additional tables*, Edinburgh: The Scottish Government.

Thomas, C. (2007) *Sociologies of Disability and Illness: Contested ideas in disability studies and medical sociology,* Basingstoke and New York: Palgrave Macmillan.

Thorvaldsdottir, T. (2007) 'Equal opportunities for all: Intersectionality as a theoretical tool to move equality policies forward', Paper presented in Reykjav'ik, Iceland, 16 March 2007, www.issa.nl/members/member_docs/ESJ_files/at_docs/add_pdfs/Intersectionality.pdf.

Thygesen, H. (2009) *Technology and Good Dementia Care. A study of technology and ethics in everyday care practice,* PhD dissertation, University of Oslo, Oslo: Oslo Academic Press.

Thygesen, H. and Moser, I. (2010) 'Technology and good dementia care: an argument for an ethics-in-practice approach', in M. Schillmeier and M. Doménech (eds) *New Technologies and Emerging Spaces of Care,* London: Ashgate, pp 129–47.

Tronto, J.C. (1993) *Moral Boundaries: A political argument for an Ethic of Care,* London: Routledge.

Tronto, J.C. (2005) 'Care as the work of citizens: a modest proposal', in M. Friedman (ed) *Women and Citizenship,* New York: Oxford University Press, pp 130–45.

Tronto, J. (2007) 'Book Review: Carol C. Gould, *Globalizing Democracy and Human Rights*', *The Good Society,* vol 16, no 2, pp 38–40.

Tronto, J. (2010) 'Creating caring institutions: politics, plurality and purpose', *Ethics and Social Welfare,* vol 4, no 2, pp 158–71.

Tronto, J. (2013) *Caring Democracy. Markets, Equality and Justice,* New York and London: New York University Press.

Twigg, J. (2006) *The Body in Health and Social Care,* Basingstoke: Palgrave.

UNFPA (2011) *State of the World Population 2011,* New York: United Nations Population Fund.

UN (UN General Assembly) (2000) *United Nations Millennium Declaration, Resolution Adopted by the General Assembly,* 18 September, A/RES/55/2, www.refworld.org/docid/3b00f4ea3.html.

United Nations (2009) *State of the World's Indigenous Peoples. Economic and social affairs,* New York: United Nations.

United Nations (2010) *Human Rights Minority Rights: International Standards and Guidance for Implementation,* New York: United Nations.

Verkerk, M. (1999) 'A care perspective on coercion and autonomy', *Bioethics,* vol 13, nos 3–4, pp 358–68.

Vila, L.J.C. (2004) *Remittances: Third world's 2nd biggest source of capital,* www.ifad.org/media/news/2004/091204_1.htm.

Visvanathan, S. (2005) 'Knowledge, justice and democracy', in M. Leach, I. Scoones and B. Wynne (eds) *Science and Citizens: Globalization and the Challenge of Engagement*, London: Zed Books.

Vojak, C. (2009) 'Choosing language: Social service framing and social justice', *British Journal of Social Work*, vol 39, pp 936–49.

Walker, A. (ed) (1996) *The New Generational Contract: Intergenerational relations, old age and welfare*, London: UCL Press.

Walker, M.U. (2006) *Moral Repair: Reconstructing Moral Relations after Wrongdoing*, New York: Cambridge University Press.

Walker, M.U. (2007) *Moral Understandings. A Feminist Study in Ethics*, Oxford: Oxford University Press.

Walker, R. (1990) *Ka Whawhai Tonu Matou – Struggle Without End*, Auckland: Penguin.

Ward, A. (2006a) 'Models of "ordinary" and "special" daily living: matching residential care to the mental-health needs of looked after children', *Child and Family Social Work*, vol 11, pp 336–46.

Ward, L., Barnes, M. and Gahagan, B. (2012) *Older People and Wellbeing. A report of a participatory research project*, Brighton: University of Brighton, Age UK Brighton and Hove.

Ward, L. and Gahagan, B. (2010) 'Crossing the divide between theory and practice: research and an ethic of care', *Ethics and Social Welfare*, vol 4, no 2, pp 210–16.

Ward, N.J. (2005) 'Social exclusion and mental wellbeing: lesbian experiences', PhD thesis, University of Birmingham.

Ward, N.J. (2009) 'Social exclusion, social identity and social work: analysing social exclusion from a material discursive perspective', *Social Work Education*, vol 28, pp 3, 237–52.

Ward, N. (2011) 'Care ethics and carers with learning disabilities: a challenge to dependence and paternalism', *Ethics and Social Welfare*, vol 5, no 2, pp 168–80.

Webb, S. (2006) *Social Work in a Risk Society: Social and policy perspectives*, Basingstoke: Palgrave.

Weedon, C. (1999) *Feminism, Theory and the Politics of Difference*, Oxford: Blackwell.

Wetherell, M. (2008) 'Subjectivity or psycho-discursive practices? Investigating complex intersectional identities', *Subjectivity*, vol 22, pp 73–81.

Whangapirita, L., Awatere, S. and Nikora, L.W. (2003) *A Review of Environment Waikato Iwi Environment Management Plans*, Environment Waikato Internal Series 2004/01 (Technical Report 2), Hamilton, New Zealand: Environment Waikato Regional Council.

WHO (World Health Organization) (2002) *Active Ageing: A policy framework*, Geneva: WHO.

WHO (2006) *Antiretroviral Therapy for HIV Infection in Adults and Adolescents: Recommendations for a Public Health Approach 2006 Revision*, Geneva: World Health Organization.

WHO (2009) *Life Expectancy by World Bank Income Group*, http://apps. who.int/gho/data/view.main.700.

WHO (2010) *Antiretroviral Therapy for HIV Infection in Adults and Adolescents: Recommendations for a Public Health Approach 2010 Revision*, Geneva: World Health Organization.

WHO (2011) 'WHO Global Code of Practice on the International Recruitment of Health Personnel', www.who.int/hrh/migration/ code/full_text/en/index.html.

WHO (2014) 'CD4+ T-Cell counting Technology', www.who.int/ diagnostics_laboratory/faq/cd4/en/ (accessed 24 September 2014).

Wiggan, G. (2011) 'Introduction: Power, privilege and the socio-cultural dimensions of education', in G. Wiggan (ed) *Power, Privilege and Education: Pedagogy, curriculum and student outcomes*, New York: Nova Science Publications.

Wiggins, D. (1991) 'Categorical requirements: Kant and Hume on the idea of duty', *Monist*, vol 74, no 1, pp 83–106.

Wilkins, D. (2012) 'Ethical dilemmas in social work practice with disabled people: The use of physical restraint', *Journal of Intellectual Disabilities*, vol 16, pp 127–33.

Willems, D. and Pols, J. (2010) 'Goodness! The empirical turn in health care ethics', *Medische Antropologie*, vol 22, no 1, pp 161–70.

Williams, F. (2001) 'In and beyond New Labour: Towards a new political ethics of care', *Critical Social Policy*, vol 21, no 4, pp 467–93.

Williams, F. (2002) 'The presence of feminism in the future of welfare', *Economy and Society*, vol 31, no 4, 502–19.

Williams, F. (2004a) *Rethinking Families*, London: Calouste Gulbenkian Foundation.

Williams, F. (2004b) 'What matters is what works: why every child matters to New Labour. Commentary on the DfES Green Paper *Every Child Matters*', *Critical Social Policy*, vol 24, no 3, pp 406–27.

Williams, F. (2010) 'Review article. Migration and care: themes, concepts and challenges', *Social Policy and Society*, vol 9, no 3, pp 385–96.

Williams, F. (2012) 'Care relations and public policy: social justice claims and social investment frames', *Families, Relationships and Societies*, vol 1, no 1, pp 103–19.

Williams, F. and Gavanas, A. (2008) 'The Intersection of child care regimes and migration regimes: a three-country study', in H. Lutz (ed) *Migration and Domestic Work: a European Perspective on a Global Theme*, Aldershot: Ashgate.

Williams, P. (2009) *Social Work with People with Learning Difficulties*, 2nd edn, Exeter: Learning Matters.

Willis, P., Ward, N.J. and Fish, J. (2011) 'Searching for LGBT carers: mapping a research agenda in social work and social care', *British Journal of Social Work,* vol 41, pp 1304–20.

Wilson, J. (2014) 'Model villages in the neoliberal era: the Millennium Development Goals and the colonization of everyday life', *Journal of Peasant Studies*, vol 41, no 1, pp 107–25.

Wilson, P., Kendall, S. and Brooks, F. (2007) 'The Expert Patients Programme: a paradox of patient empowerment and medical dominance', *Health and Social Care in the Community*, vol 15, no 5, pp 426–38.

Wiskow, C. (2005) *Management of International Health Worker Migration: Instruments on Ethical Recruitment and Other Policy Options*, unpublished mimeo, Geneva: WHO.

Wolin, S.S. (2008) *Democracy Incorporated: Managed Democracy and the Specter of Inverted Totalitarianism,* Princeton, NJ: Princeton University Press.

World Bank (2013) 'Developing countries to receive over $410 billion remittances in 2013', Washington, DC: World Bank.

Yea-huey, S. (2007) 'Full responsibility with partial citizenship: immigrant wives in Taiwan', *Social Policy & Administration*, vol 41, pp 179–96.

Yeates, N. (2004) 'A dialogue with "global care chain" analysis: nurse migration in the Irish context', *Feminist Review*, vol 77, no 1, pp 79–95.

Yong, A. (2007) *Theology and Down Syndrome: Reimagining disability in late modernity*, Waco, TX: Baylor University Press.

Young, I.M. (1997) 'Asymmetrical reciprocity: On moral respect, wonder and enlarged thought', *Constellations*, vol 3, no 3, pp 340–63.

Young, I.M. (2011) *Responsibility for Justice*, New York: Oxford University Press.

Yuval Davis, N. (2006a) 'Intersectionality and feminist politics', *European Journal of Women's Studies*, vol 13, no 3, pp 193–209.

Yuval Davis, N. (2006b) 'Belonging and the politics of belonging', *Patterns of Prejudice*, vol 40, no 3, pp 197–214.

Yuval Davis, N. (2011) *The Politics of Belonging: Intersectional contestations*, California: Sage.

Zontini, E. (2013) 'Care arrangements for transnational migrant elders: between family, community and the state', in C. Rodgers and S. Weller (eds) *Critical Approaches to Care. Understanding caring relations, identities and cultures*, London: Routledge.

Index

O

O'Carroll, A.D. 73
Omolade, B. 88
Orme, J. 4
Our Bodies Ourselves 47–8

P

Paradza, G.G. 142, 146
past injustices 41, 70, 77–80
Peacock, D. 140
Pease, B. 87, 94
Pedwell, C. 102
peer support 156–63
people living with HIV (PLHA) *see* HIV
    care
personal experiences 236–8
personal responsibility 49–50
personalisation of care 10
Phillips, A. 48
photographic representation of disability
    179–93, 238
physical presence and care 38–9
physical restraint, use of
    acceptability of 200
    alternatives to 197–8
    and care ethics 198–204
    context of 196–8
    definition of 197
    effects of 197–8
    experiences of 200–4
    justification for 200–1
    research project 195, 200–2
    and rights-based discourse 199
    and violence 203–4
PLHA (people living with HIV) *see* HIV
    care
Plumwood, V. 85–7
Pollak, S. 211–12
Pols, J. 17
poststructuralism 57, 58, 60–7
power
    and AIDS carers 144–8
    empowerment 49–52, 153
    and identity 59, 60, 63
    and interdependence 153–4
    and intersectionality 60, 63
    and people with intellectual disabilities
        182, 190
    and privileged irresponsibility 6, 77–8,
        83–5
    and self-care 47–52
    and use of physical restraint 203
privilege
    definition of 83–4
    and dualism 85–7
privileged irresponsibility
    in care provision 89–91

and colonisation 77–8, 87–8
concept of 6, 77, 85
definition of privilege 83–4
and dualism 85–7
and gender 90–1, 92–3
and indigenous cultures 77–8
and renewal 236
resistance to 91–4
and social connection model 93–4
in South Africa 85–91
protection 6, 189, 220, 222–3, 224
public health 50, 53–4
Pulcini, E. 41, 42

Q

queer communities 63–4

R

radical exclusion 86
Rakusen, J. 48
reciprocity 16, 33
    and carers with intellectual disabilities
        166–9, 176–7
    and collective care 35, 37
    and indigenous cultures 75
    and telecare 115
    see also interdependency
recognition 126–8, 131, 138
Reik, T. 100
relational autonomy 112, 153, 160, 163
relational ontology 3–4
relationships of care 14–16
    and attentiveness 38, 97, 169–71, 173,
        177, 191–2, 224–6, 230
    and caring democracy 28
    children as carers 151–2, 154–6, 157
    and competence 173–4, 226–7, 230
    in day care centres 125–6, 131–8
    and dialogue 238–40
    and documentation 135–6
    and empathy 99, 102–6, 153
    fluidity of 33
    and gender imbalance 140–1, 143–4,
        160, 161, 162, 163
    at global level 22–3
    and identity 59, 65–8
    and International Child Development
        Programme 96, 103–5
    and intimacy 39–40
    and Māori culture 73–5
    and men's role 140, 143–4, 145, 160
    and medical migrants 208–9
    mother-child relationship 32, 147,
        154–6
    multidimensionality of 33–5
    and networks and collectives 35–7
    and peer support 156–63